610.73 MAS

Visit our website

to find out about other books from Churc
and our sister imprints in Harcourt Healt

Register free at
www.harcourt-international.com

and you will get

- the latest information on new books, journals and electronic products in your chosen subject areas

- the choice of e-mail or post alerts or both, when there are any new books in your chosen areas

- news of special offers and promotions

- information about products from all Harcourt Health Sciences imprints including Baillière Tindall, Churchill Livingstone, Mosby and W. B. Saunders

You will also find an easily searchable catalogue, online ordering, information on our extensive list of journals...and much more!

Visit the Harcourt Health Sciences' website today!

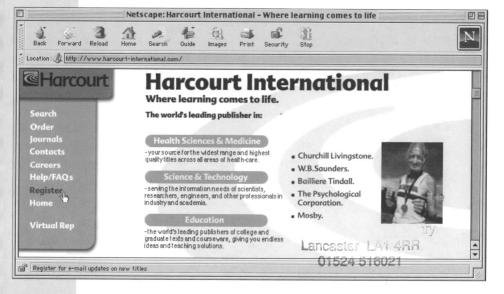

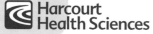

Developing New Clinical Roles

For Churchill Livingstone:

Senior Commissioning Editor: Jacqueline Curthoys
Project Development Manager: Karen Gilmour
Project Manager: Derek Robertson
Design Direction: George Ajayi

Developing New Clinical Roles
A Guide for Health Professionals

Edited by

Abigail Masterson MN, BSc, RN, PGCEA
Director, Abi Masterson Consulting Ltd, Southampton, UK

Debra Humphris PhD, MA, DipN(Lon), RN, RNT
Senior Research Fellow, Health Care Evaluation Unit, St George's Hospital Medical School, London, UK

Foreword by

John Rogers
Formerly Deputy Director of Human Resources, NHS Executive, England

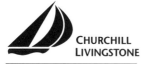
CHURCHILL
LIVINGSTONE

EDINBURGH LONDON NEW YORK PHILADELPHIA ST LOUIS SYDNEY TORONTO 2000

CHURCHILL LIVINGSTONE
An imprint of Harcourt Publishers Limited

© Harcourt Publishers Limited 2000

 is a registered trademark of Harcourt Publishers Limited

The rights of Debra Humphris and Abigail Masterson to be identified as editors of this work have been asserted by them in accordance with the Copyright, Designs and Patents Act 1988

First published 2000

ISBN 0443 07071 7

British Library Cataloguing in Publication Data
A catalogue record for this book is available from the British Library

Library of Congress Cataloging in Publication Data
A catalog record for this book is available from the Library of Congress

The
publisher's
policy is to use
paper manufactured
from sustainable forests

Printed in China

Contents

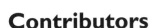

Contributors

Ailsa Cameron BA (Hons), MSc
Research Fellow, School for Policy Studies, University of Bristol

Nicola Davey BPharm, MPhil, MRPharms
Freelance consultant on research and policy developments for pharmacy and the wider health agenda in England, Scotland and Wales

Lesley Doyal MSc, BA
Professor of Health and Social Care, School for Policy Studies, University of Bristol

Dr Ann Drury MBBS, FRCR
Practising clinician and Chair of the Junior Doctors' Task Force, South Thames Region

Sarah Fisher MSc, BSc, RN
Deputy Director of Nursing, University College London Hospitals NHS Trust, London

Tina Funnell
Independent consultant on patient issues, Chair of the Consumer Health Information Centre and Organising Secretary of the Health Coalition Initiative

Debra Humphris PhD, MA, DipN(Lond), RN, RNT
Senior Research Fellow, Health Care Evaluation Unit, St George's Hospital Medical School, London

Abigail Masterson MN, BSc, RN, PGCEA
Director, Abi Masterson Consulting Ltd, Southampton

Anne Palmer MA, BEd(Hons), RN, RM, RNT
Education Consultant working in the NHS and Director of Postgraduate Studies, Centre for Community Care and Primary Health, University of Westminster

Geraldine Walters PhD, MBA, BSc, RN
Assistant Director of Nursing, NHS Executive, London Region

Foreword

This book could not have been written a decade or so ago. A statement of the obvious, for certain, but it is worth reminding ourselves how quickly change has taken place since the mid-1980s. At that time, talk of changes to professional boundaries, non-hierarchical teams, specialist practice (outside the medical profession) and interprofessional education was largely the preserve of consenting adults in private. Yet today a Secretary of State for Health can say 'we need to modernise fossilised ways of working which owe more to the NHS of 1948 than the world of the 21st century. That means breaking down barriers between professions so that patients get more holistic, more streamlined care' (Alan Milburn, November 1999), without causing the ornaments to fall off the mantelpiece.

This book explains some of the influences behind the rapid change in professional roles and practice; gives specific examples of change in practice and advice on how to develop and manage new roles; and, importantly, approaches the difficult question of evaluation. For it has to be said that there is still a great paucity of hard evidence about the effect of changes to roles and skillmix on the quality, outcome or cost of care. This will be one of the challenges for the first decade of this century, along with the implications for professional regulatory machinery, education and the medico-legal framework.

My overriding impression of the last decade is that role changes, even where sparked by external factors such as technology or junior doctors' issues, have been largely driven by a patient-centred perception of the delivery of health care. True, this has mostly been managers' and professionals' views of a patient focus – but I suspect the role changes of the next decade or two will be driven by a much more explicit involvement of patients and clients in designing the delivery of services. We are only at the beginning of a long road.

For anyone who wants to make sense of the developments of the last decade and to gain some insight into where we may be headed, I commend this book.

John Rogers,
Formerly **Deputy Director of Human Resources,**
NHS Executive, England
2000

Introduction

Debra Humphris   Abigail Masterson

Throughout the health-care system the traditional boundaries between professional groups are becoming increasingly blurred in response to local service needs and national policy objectives. Many new clinical roles have been created that are beginning to redefine the boundaries between medicine, nursing and the health-care professions (HCPs). Many of these new role developments are linked to specific policies affecting medical work and education such as the 'New deal' which, along with pressure from patient groups, developments from within the professions themselves, technological developments and demographic changes, have impacted on the traditional division of labour in health care.

The origins of this book lie in the work we have been involved in for the United Kingdom Central Council for Nursing, Midwifery and Health Visiting on the regulation of specialist, advanced and higher-level practice, the Department of Health (England) on researching new role developments in nursing and the HCPs and in working with the Regional Task Forces set up to manage the reduction in junior doctors' hours as a consequence of the 'New deal'. The insights gained from these experiences provoked us to commission authors from a variety of professional backgrounds to examine the development of new clinical roles in nursing and the HCPs.

Our intention in the production of this book is to provide a comprehensive and thought-provoking text for practitioners, managers and policy-makers in nursing, medicine and the HCPs regarding the development of new clinical roles. It offers a broad range of perspectives on the phenomenon of new clinical role development coupled with practical ideas to promote sensitive, appropriate and sustainable development. Each chapter is capable of standing alone while also contributing to the structure of the book as a whole. The examples and case studies used are not meant to be definitive; rather they represent parts of an evolving debate. Their fundamental purpose is to act as a resource, to stimulate thinking, generate debate and encourage further local and national exploration of the issues raised.

Ailsa Cameron, in Chapter 1, discusses the socio-political context within which this new role development is occurring. The drivers for new role development, such as the 'New deal' for junior doctors, waiting list initiatives and changes in the delivery of health services such as day surgery and the reduction in lengths of stay are explored. The implications of these developments for the position of medicine within the health-care system and the scope of practice within nursing and the HCPs are considered. Technology, demography, health needs and the shape and structure of the future health-care workforce are also critically examined. The importance of health and social policy in determining new role developments is highlighted. Cameron concludes that in view of the increasing pace of change, the blurring of professional boundaries is only likely to continue. She reminds us, however, that new does not necessarily mean better and that change merely for the sake of it should be avoided. Her analysis highlights the importance of joint planning and mutual respect across the health professions at local and national levels.

New role development in primary care is examined from the perspective of community pharmacy. In Chapter 2 Nicola Davey looks at the history of community pharmacy and at the statutory requirements of the profession and their impact on the role of the pharmacist and the services that are currently provided. Factors affecting role development such as qualifications, skill mix, multiprofessional contact, remuneration packages and the 1990 reforms are reviewed. The nature and diverse roles of the pharmacy-related professional organisations are examined in relation to regulation, advisory functions, training and negotiation. Emerging models of practice are reviewed in light of the changing roles of pharmacists and other caring professions. Finally the opportunities and challenges, both short- and long-term, are considered. Davey concludes that the 21st century holds many promises for pharmacists and many more for primary care if the health professions begin working together in a more complementary and holistic way to deliver truly patient-focused care.

The current professional interest in the development of evidence-based practice reflects the Government's aim that health-care interventions should stem from a sound research base and be subject to evaluation of their effectiveness. In Chapter 3, Sarah Fisher discusses how practitioners in new clinical roles can promote the development of a practice environment that is conducive to implementing evidence-based practice. She clarifies how practitioners in new roles should access, appraise and integrate research evidence in their area of practice and share the findings with patients. The area of practice used to illustrate the key points raised throughout the chapter is that of cardiac care, a specialty in which a range of new roles is gradually being defined across a range of professions. Fisher argues that practitioners in new roles have a responsibility to develop services based on sound evidence and audit to demonstrate the benefits of their role for patients and to realise improvements in care.

In Chapter 4 Anne Palmer explores personal and professional development. She argues that practitioners working in new clinical roles need to become adult learners who are confident enough to challenge current assumptions about practice. She posits that for true reflection in practice to occur such practitioners require critical thinking skills, an appreciation of portfolio-based learning approaches and the ability to seek out enabling relationships that promote their personal and professional development. Questions are raised about the current National Health Service (NHS) climate and its ability to promote learning. Palmer argues that it is necessary to promote an organisational culture that encourages curiosity, experiment and self-discovery. Such a culture should also promote individual respect and open dialogue through frameworks of professional support. Those practitioners working in new clinical roles are presented as being uniquely placed to encourage the development of such a climate.

Geraldine Walters, in Chapter 5, examines the ways in which new roles need to develop in order to make a strategic impact on the provision of health care in the future. She considers the background to new role developments and suggests the infrastructure required to support these roles and achieve their maximum potential. She reviews existing examples of models of specialist practice in nursing and explores their associated tensions. She illustrates the difficulties involved in managing the development and contribution of new clinical roles within the NHS. Specific reference is made to 'The new NHS: modern, dependable', recruitment and retention, professional/service tensions, education, career structures and remuneration.

Ailsa Cameron and Lesley Doyal, in Chapter 6, review new role development across the professions. They draws on research evidence from the 'Exploring new roles in practice' project to illustrate the experiences of members of the HCPs working in new roles. The chapter identifies some of the similarities between the experiences of HCPs and nurses as well as the differences related to the size and representation of these professions within acute care. They note that the roles they discuss have played an important part in demonstrating the potential contribution of health-care professionals to new patterns of health care. At the same time, however, they raise important questions about current professional and service boundaries, about specialisation and genericism and about the future not just of traditional HCP career structures but even of the professions themselves.

'If patients don't change health care, who will?' Tina Funnell asks this simple yet powerful question in her introduction to Chapter 7. Using her own experiences spanning over 20 years as a consumer representative in health care she challenges many of the existing traditional models of care. Starting from the premise that patients are first and foremost human beings with human hopes and needs, not simply diseases with a person attached, she explains that increasingly patients want to take a more active role in determining the nature of their health care. Funnell illustrates how, in trying to balance the dimensions of cost, quality and access to ensure optimum outcomes, the interests and needs of patients are still too often obscured. She argues that to change the health service fundamentally into a truly patient-centred service, patients' views need to be valued, respected, understood and acted upon. Funnell reminds us that new role developments in all professions should start from patients and their needs and as such may require revolutions in existing structures, services and even professions.

Chapter 8 reflects the changes which have been taking place in medical education and the profession itself. Ann Drury explains that the catalyst for changes in medical education was the Department of Health's introduction of the 'New deal on junior doctors' hours' in 1991, the so-called 'Calman report', which introduced structured training and education to enable appointment to consultant grade. There is often limited understanding by professional groups of how other professions train and progress in their careers. This chapter attempts to demystify many of the changes that have taken place within the medical profession that have had significant consequences for the other professional groups in health care.

In Chapter 9 we review and critique the development of new roles and argue that evaluation is key in the process of new role development. We highlight the lack of outcome studies to date and the methodological challenges that researching such roles poses. Using a case study from radiography we highlight the complexities involved in developing rigorous evaluations. We advocate the development of evaluation partnerships consisting of researchers, human resource staff, managers, consumers and practitioners, to draw out the practical and cost-effective implications of such evaluations for future workforce and service development.

In the final chapter we introduce an international dimension to these debates. We re-examine the forces for change such as consumerism, primary care, technology, the inevitability of innovation in practice and the evolving relationship between the needs and demands of health-care roles and delivery. We then reflect specifically on the UK parliamentary health committee's recommendations for the wider workforce in the NHS. We argue that the health professions are faced with a stark choice as to whether they deploy their resources to defend their existing boundaries or embrace the changes within the global context of health care.

The emergence of new clinical roles has provided each of the health professions with opportunities to review its contribution to health care and to the multiprofessional teams it works in to deliver health services. We welcome this scrutiny as a necessary aspect of modernising health care. We believe the development of new clinical roles can be a potent force for truly patient-focused care if carried out in a structured manner and as part of strategic service and workforce development. Throughout the text the key message for all health professionals is to learn about and respect the contributions made by others.

The development of new clinical roles raises countless professional issues and offers tremendous opportunities to redefine roles, autonomy and ultimately status. In the future we should not be creating new roles without a systematic framework of evaluation. So whilst new roles will constantly be needed so too will the robust and rigorous evaluation of such developments. To ensure practitioners in new clinical roles can contribute meaningfully to service developments they require a political and organisational awareness. In this way they may be able to balance the constant tension between the ever-present task of finding workforce solutions to service problems and developing and changing professional roles in a systematic and coherent manner for the benefit of patients.

New role developments in context

Ailsa Cameron

Introduction

There can be little doubt that UK health care has changed markedly over the last two decades (Ham 1992). Many commentators have focused upon the drive towards a primary care led NHS and the introduction of quasi markets as evidence of this change (Nettleton 1997, Ranade 1997). But one of the most interesting trends has been the proliferation of new clinical roles for nurses and the health-care professions (HCPs) in primary and secondary care and the subsequent debate about the nature of specialist and advanced practice. Although it may be tempting for nurses and HCPs to believe that such developments are professionally driven, it is the central contention of this chapter that these changes have occurred in response to a variety of external and internal factors. This chapter aims to explore these role developments and place them firmly in a context of change within the health care system.

In order to analyse the development of new roles for nurses and HCPs we need to look outside the professions and take into account the wider context of the health care system, its policy context. Practitioners may not always see the relevance of such an analysis. However exploration of the interaction between changes in policy and the evolution of new roles will help nurses and HCPs proactively manage future developments, in particular, their boundaries with other professions. For example nursing in the United Kingdom has always been influenced by the views of government and dominant groups in the policy making process (Robinson 1992). However, it appears that the profession has often been caught unawares by crucial developments that have driven significant changes within the health-care system (Cameron & Masterson 2000). The debate about the development and even the desirability of nurse practitioner roles came after their introduction into acute and primary care services. As a result the profession was in a much weaker position to manage and control the development (United Kingdom Central Council for Nursing, Midwifery and Health Visiting 1998). More recently the announcement by the Prime Minister of the creation of a 'super nurse' appeared to surprise those involved in the UKCC review of higher level practice (1998). This illustrates a lack of co-ordination between key players in the regulation and development of the profession and those at the centre of the policy process.

Health and social policy is therefore an important area of study for all health professionals, whether they see their role as 'hands on' or strategic (Baker 1996). Studying policy can enable practitioners to gain greater insight into developments within their profession. It can also provide nurses and HCPs with the tools to assess future policy changes and thus exert influence over the course of events. Crucially, the voices of nurses and HCPs need to be heard in health and social policy debates. Without their involvement, decisions about the way health care is provided and about the composition of the health care workfore will be taken without full consideration of the profesional issues (Gough et al 1994).

Nursing: a case study

One of the more striking changes within the NHS over the last decade has been the increase in new nursing roles. Before examining the external factors that have led to the creation of new nursing roles I will first consider the forces for change from within the nursing profession.

George Castledine (professor of nursing and UKCC Council Member) has argued that the development of clinical nurse specialist roles and advanced practice nursing in the United Kingdom results from four critical influences: specialist hospitals and specialist health care; the 'Manchester School'; the RCN; and the political and professional regulatory processes (Castledine 1994). Let us now explore these drivers for change in more detail.

Specialist hospitals and specialist health care

There is little doubt that health-care roles have developed to meet the needs of patients requiring specialist treatment. Ham identifies the importance of the 'Calman–Hine report on the organisation and delivery of cancer services' as a catalyst for change in the way health-care professionals work together as well as leading to the creation of designated breast surgeons and colorectal surgeons (Ham et al 1997). This initiative has undoubtedly also encouraged the development of new nursing roles. Similarly, advances in technology, pharmacology and medical practice have resulted in a plethora of new nursing roles such as breast-care specialists, nurse counsellors and chemotherapy nurse specialists. Developments in nursing knowledge and practice have hastened these developments, but as Castledine points out, many of these roles originate from the need to have technically competent nurses to perform paramedical procedures rather than from the development of clinical nursing practice. I will return to the impact of technological developments on new role development later in the chapter when external drivers for change are discussed.

The 'Manchester School'

Castledine's assertion that the 'Manchester School' (a group of influential nurses who studied on one of the early Masters in Nursing programmes at Manchester University in the 1980s) has been crucial in the development of specialist and advanced practice nursing is an interesting although somewhat narrow interpretation. Indeed there was a wave of creative and developmental energy in the 1980s that was crucial to the advancement of nursing practice, but much of the impetus came from grass roots initiatives as well as from academic and strategic initiatives. For example, the impact of the Radical

Midwives Group on the development of women-centred and midwife-led maternity services (Department of Health 1993a) is an impressive testament to the ability of grass roots practitioners to shape policy and practice.

However, the 'Manchester School' certainly influenced the 'Nursing development' movement that flourished in the 1980s. This movement came to prominence on the back of initiatives such as the 'Nursing process', which was intended to be not only a system of documentation, but also a way of illustrating the value of nursing and its unique contribution to health care. During the late 1980s the nursing development movement appeared to have had a significant influence on the policy and professional agenda. For example, the Department of Health (DoH) supported the establishment of nursing development units as a means of encouraging excellence in practice. The self-confidence of the profession was manifest in the empowering rhetoric of primary nursing and the legislative support for educational change (UKCC 1986, Salvage & Wright 1995). This wave of professional optimism was probably significant in that it fostered a decade of professional advancement, so important to the development of specialist and advanced nursing practice.

The RCN and the influence of political and professional regulatory processes

The role of the RCN has also been important in determining the direction of nursing developments. The work of Barbara Stilwell (at that time a member of staff in the RCN's Institute of Advanced Nursing Education) has been critical in fostering the education and development of nurse practitioners, particularly those working in primary care, in the UK. One might suggest, however, that a most potent internal factor has been the influence of what Castledine called the political and professional regulatory processes, in particular the UKCC's 'The scope of professional practice' document (UKCC 1992a). Many commentators have described 'Scope' as the culmination of nursing's liberation (Paniagua 1995, Land, Mhaolrunaigh & Castledine 1996). Historically, if nurses wanted to take on duties or responsibilities that were not traditionally associated with the nursing role or covered in pre-registration education, such as intravenous drug administration or suturing, employers insisted on further training and extended role certificates for each extra 'task' (DHSS 1977). 'Scope' put the responsibility for ensuring competence firmly on the shoulders of each individual nurse by emphasising the pivotal role of his/her interpretation of his/her own professional accountability. In doing so the UKCC placed decisions about the boundaries of practice in the hands of practitioners (Redfern 1997). Nurses are now free to exercise their own judgement about the tasks they perform so long as any new role adopted does not adversely affect patient care or contravene the principles expressed in the 'Code of professional conduct' (UKCC 1992b). Both documents provided nurses, midwives and health visitors with a degree of professional autonomy which enabled them to provide innovative solutions to meet the needs of patients in a health service that is constantly changing (UKCC 1997). Without doubt such professional developments helped demolish unhelpful barriers between the health-care professions with the result that nurses could develop their roles into areas that previously were firmly within the domain of medicine.

Another important driver for change that came from within the regulatory process was the UKCC's 'Post-registration education and practice' (PREP) report published in 1994. This report, which launched a number of proposals for changing the post-registration educational structure and knowledge base of the profession, has been heralded as recognising the academic value of nurse education (Roberts-Davies et al 1998). PREP identified two further levels of practice beyond registration – specialist and advanced – clearly acknowledging and supporting the development of nursing practice and the development of new nursing roles.

Overall, UK nursing during the 1980s and early 1990s had moved towards a model of practice which promoted autonomy and accountability and allowed nursing the room to develop in new ways to meet the changing health needs of the population at large. Nurses were now better placed to develop new roles but why were those roles necessary?

The wider policy context

The UKCC noted in its document 'Scope in practice' that 'no profession is an island', suggesting that professional developments need to be seen within a broader context that acknowledges other forces for change such as the reduction in junior doctors' hours of work, 'Health of the nation' initiatives and disease management processes (UKCC 1997). The 1996 'Report of the Standing Nursing and Midwifery Advisory Committee' argued that a mature profession would use these external forces as a lever for advancement rather than simply reacting to them (Standing Nursing and Midwifery Advisory Committee (SNMAC) 1996). Unfortunately, a reactive posture has frequently been adopted. Let us now review the external drivers for change that lay behind the development of new nursing roles.

The impact of health service reform

The importance of legislation in shaping health care is beyond doubt. Less obvious perhaps is the relationship between legislation and the development of new professional roles. In this section we explain the impact of legislation intended to reform the NHS on the development of new clinical roles.

The 1990 NHS and Community Care Act

The 1990 *NHS and Community Care Act* represented a dramatic attack on the notion of centralised planning and professional control over health services in the UK. Prior to its introduction Regional Health Authorities had retained a strategic planning function over all District Health Authorities but the 1990 legislation signalled not only an end to this relationship but also a direct challenge to professional power (Ranade 1997). The 1990 reforms led to the introduction of what has become known as the internal market. The Act aimed to foster some of the qualities of competition, choice and management discipline which characterise private enterprise (Ham 1992). In essence the Act led to a split between the purchasing and providing functions of the NHS. Individual hospitals or groups of hospitals could apply for trust status. This gave them power to determine which services they would provide and the terms and conditions of employment of the staff working in them. Trusts were also given the opportunity to generate income. In other words, they were encouraged to provide responsive, market-driven services. The 1990 Act also allowed general practitioners (GPs) to apply to become fundholding practices. As such, the GPs were given a budget from their Regional Health Authority, which was weighted to reflect the needs of their population. The budget was used to contract with, or rather purchase a defined range of health-care services from any hospital that was able to meet the GPs' needs in the most efficient and cost-effective manner. The services that fundholding GPs were allowed to purchase included outpatients' services, diagnostic tests and inpatient care.

This fundamental change in the way services were purchased and provided had implications for the professions involved in delivering services. The introduction of Trusts as independent financial units forced a re-examination of the most cost-effective means of providing services, which led to initiatives such as workforce re-engineering, skill mix reviews and, in many instances, the development of new professional roles. For example, some Trusts introduced nurse-led clinics and rapid discharge programmes in an attempt to make services more efficient (Ong 1997). Other Trusts responded to these new managerial challenges by drastically reconfiguring the services they provided. There has also been a rapid increase in the prevalence of roles such as nurse anaesthetists (Audit Commission 1997), nurse endoscopists (UKCC 1997) and surgeons' assistants (Tuthill 1995). Such posts were often introduced as a means of increasing the efficiency and cost-effectiveness of services by better utilising the knowledge and experience of individual nurses.

Similarly, the growing emphasis on primary care led GPs to develop services that in the past would have been provided in hospital. Ham et al (1997) argue that GPs enjoyed growing influence as a result of their role as purchasers of health services and suggest that GPs used this influence to force change on the way health services are provided. For example, GPs could demand that the outpatient clinics and screening services they purchased from acute Trusts were delivered in the GP practice rather than in hospital, and could carry out minor surgical procedures themselves rather than refer a patient to a consultant. As a consequence therefore GPs have been able to influence the way in which individual practitioners work. The growing number of asthma nurses and diabetes specialist nurses working across the primary/secondary care interface who can prescribe within protocols for conditions such as hypertension, asthma and diabetes bears witness to this phenomenon. But it isn't just nursing that has been affected by the increasing influence of GPs. There are growing numbers of sonographers working in general practice who provide quick access to diagnostic images, a trend which marks a fundamental change to their traditional pattern of employment. Physiotherapists, occupational therapists and counsellors are also increasingly working out of GP practices or under contract to GPs and tailoring their services to the wishes of the GP.

'The new NHS: modern, dependable'

In December 1997 the new Labour Government announced its proposals for the NHS. The White Paper, 'The new NHS: modern, dependable', stated that from April 1999 Primary Care Groups (PCGs) would replace fundholding arrangements. PCGs would comprise GPs and community nurses who would work together to improve the health of the population they serve. The groups would commission health services for their population from relevant NHS Trusts and work in partnership with local authorities to ensure that primary and community health services are better integrated with social services.

This means that, despite the rhetoric of partnership, health services will continue to be configured around a division between those who commission services and those who provide them. This has implications for the nursing profession as well as for the role of individual nurses. First, the trend towards involving primary health-care workers in the commissioning of services is set to continue, with nursing being given a major role in the commissioning process. Will this herald a new managerial role for nurses or possibly the rise of a public health nurse who is a specialist in epidemiology? Indeed the White Paper explicitly stated that the Government wished to encourage and 'extend the recent developments in the roles of nurses working in acute and community services. The Government is committed to encouraging and supporting the development of nursing practice in these ways' (DoH 1997)'

The second important trend that will have an impact on nursing and HCPs is the continued emphasis on informed commissioning and clinical governance which will require all professional groups to audit their clinical practice. Successful commissioning requires informed decision-making, which in turn requires detailed information. As a result, evidence-based practice will continue to be regarded as the only acceptable mode of operation in health and social care. All professions will need to articulate and justify their contribution to health care. The new clinical roles that have developed over the past decade will not be exempt from this trend (Humphris 1999). Indeed it is possible that this trend will be particularly important for those roles that transcend professional boundaries, whether they be at the nursing/medicine interface or the nursing/HCP interface. Evidence will be required to support the advancement of individual professions, particularly if it is at the expense of another profession.

The impact of government initiatives on the development of new roles

As discussed in the introduction to this chapter the shape of services and the remit of those working within them owe as much to the operationalisation of particular government initiatives as they do to legislation. To illustrate this point I will consider two highly publicised government initiatives that have encouraged the development of new roles for nurses as well as for other health-care professionals.

Waiting list initiatives

During the late 1980s and early 1990s the issue of waiting lists became a potent symbol of what many believed to be a policy of neglect towards the NHS. As a result of growing public criticism, the Conservative Government announced plans to reduce waiting lists as a way of cosmetically improving services without dealing with the issue of chronic underfunding. Central government issued guidance to health authorities indicating that no patient should wait more than 2 years for admission to hospital. One hundred new consultant posts were created to help achieve this and £33 million was made available during 1990/91 to tackle this issue (Ham 1992). The 'Patient's charter' (Department of Health 1991b) consolidated the initiative and gave patients the right to be seen within 2 years.

Each Trust developed its own strategies to reduce waiting lists. Some used the extra funding to open operating theatres and day surgery units at the weekend in an effort to increase levels of activity. Other Trusts used the extra money to fund the development of new roles. At many Trusts, nursing and therapy roles in outpatient clinics were expanded to free up surgeons so that they could spend more time in theatre. For example, orthopaedic physiotherapy practitioner posts have been created to work as part of the diagnostic team for benign musculoskeletal cases. These practitioners take patients directly off a consultant's waiting list who are thought unlikely to require surgical intervention. They can request and interpret investigations such as X-rays and scans and can plan treatment and management, including referral of the patient to other services. Pre-operative assessment roles were also created for nurses as a means of making services more efficient and patient-friendly. The skill mix in theatres was reviewed with the result that nurses have become more involved in the process of surgery as the emergence of nurse anaesthetists and clinician's assistant roles demonstrates (English 1997). These new health-care roles often included work that traditionally would have been carried out by doctors: for example, full clerking and pre-surgical work.

Waiting list initiatives have had and will continue to have major implications for the nursing and health-care professions. In November 1997 the new Labour Government announced extra funding to support renewed attempts to reduce waiting lists in line with their pre-election manifesto promises (NHS Executive 1997). As part of this initiative, regionally based task forces were established to deliver local solutions to long waiting lists and encourage the spread of good practice. The Government also created a National Waiting List Action Team which reports monthly to ministers on progress. Nursing and HCP leaders need to be strategically involved in such initiatives to ensure their opinions will inform efforts to shorten waiting lists. This would seem essential if new clinical roles are to be developed to reduce lists. If these professions do not take part in strategic management of this and other initiatives they run the risk of merely watching others shape their futures.

The 'New deal' – junior doctors' hours

Another initiative which deserves attention because of its impact on the practice of nursing and HCPs and the development of new clinical roles is the ongoing programme to reduce the hours worked by junior doctors and to reduce the contribution of doctors in training to service provision in the NHS (NHS Management Executive 1991; Department of Health 1993b). In 1991 the Government directed that employers should ensure that as soon as practicable no doctor in training should have to work longer than 83 hours a week. The maximum was then to fall to 72 hours a week by the end of 1994 for doctors working in posts that were described as 'hard-pressed'. By the end of 1996, no junior doctor was supposed to be contracted to work more than 56 hours a week (Department of Health 1991a). This measure was likely to affect the supply of junior doctors throughout the NHS as well as exacerbating shortages of junior doctors already apparent in areas such as accident and emergency and paediatrics. The Government therefore urged employers to make best use of the skills of nurses and HCPs to help reduce workloads and hours of junior doctors.

To enable this reduction, the Government allocated money to each NHS region to fund new developments. Some regions invested their 'task-force' money in the development of new clinical roles, often in nursing, to reduce junior doctors' hours. For example, Trent Region used £500 000 of its task-force money to pump-prime a raft of new nursing roles to fill gaps left by junior doctors (Murray et al 1995). Similarly, the task force in the South and West Region funded four innovative clinical nursing roles as part of their response to this policy drive. Many of the new roles funded under such schemes were developed within surgical specialties and involved the establishment of nurse-led services such as pre-operative clinics in orthopaedics and ear, nose and throat departments. There were also new posts in medical specialties such as night nurse practitioner posts and medical admissions nurse specialists. Evaluations suggest that these new roles strengthen continuity of care and reduce the intensity of junior doctors' workloads even if they may not reduce their hours (Doyal et al 1998). However, as much of the literature about these new roles is descriptive with little analysis of outcome it is unclear whether these developments have been beneficial to patients and staff.

Much has been written about the negative and positive implications for nursing and HCPs of the reduction in junior doctors' hours. The negative view implies that nurses and HCPs have had to pick up tasks that junior doctors no longer had the time or inclination to do. The positive view identifies an opportunity for these professions to increase their contribution to patient care by developing into new areas. Whatever one's view about the developments it is doubtful whether they could have happened without the introduction of the Scope of Professional Practice (UKCC 1992a), which allowed nurses to extend their work remit and take on tasks that traditionally would have been carried out by junior doctors.

Both examples demonstrate how nursing and HCP practice has developed in response to external factors, but it is debatable whether nursing and HCP leaders have played an equal part with medical colleagues in forming these initiatives. Had they played a strategic role then greater consideration might have been given to developing a more coherent and systematic approach to education and the assessment of competence required to underpin such new roles. Instead it appears that new roles have often developed in an ad hoc and incremental manner without parallel assessment of performance. Dowling et al (1996), in relation to nursing, point out the crucial importance of joint planning between the UKCC, RCN, General Medical Council and the medical Royal Colleges so that both professions develop joint responses to government initiatives to enable them to move forward together in a proactive manner.

It is important to emphasise that it was not only nurses who filled gaps left by junior doctors. Shortages of doctors in radiology have led to the extension of traditional radiography roles, thus allowing radiographers to give intravenous injections, barium enemas and in some instances to report on images. Physiotherapists have also been active in developing specialist roles, for example, in rheumatology, physiotherapy practitioners are undertaking work that once was done by junior doctors.

Changes in the delivery of health services

The manner in which health care is delivered is in part determined by external factors – that is, factors outside the control of the health professions. This section considers the impact of technological change on the way health care is delivered.

Warner & Riley define health technology as the 'drugs, devices, and medical and surgical procedures of healthcare and the systems in which such clinical technologies are provided' (Warner & Riley 1994, p. 13). Interestingly, other commentators including the NHS Health Technology Assessment programme have adopted a broader definition in which new clinical roles themselves can be considered to be technology. Whether we use the term 'technology' to refer to things or people, it has certainly had a significant influence on health-care practice and has fostered changes in the personnel delivering clinical services. For example, the development of nurse-run minor injuries centres has been supported by the advent of video conferencing techniques which allow instant access to medical teams based in other hospitals, possibly working in different parts of the country or even in different countries. Technological developments have also allowed other workers to develop the scope of their profession. Developments in radiographic practices have enabled sonographers to undertake intra-operative ultrasounds and become part of the theatre team.

I will now consider the impact of growth in day surgery and reductions in length of hospital stay on development of new professional roles.

Day surgery

One of the more profound changes in the way in which health-care services are delivered in recent years has been the growing number of patients under-going day surgery. Day surgery accounts for almost 60% of all operations and has almost trebled in the last decade to nearly 3 million cases in 1996–7 (Moore 1998). Many conditions that used to require hospital admission can now be successfully treated as day cases – for example, hernia repair and removal of benign growths. Technological and pharmacological advances and developments in miniaturisation have supported this expansion in day surgery and non-invasive therapies. Further technological advances are likely to expand the types of condition deemed appropriate for day surgery. Such developments are likely to have implications for those professions who provide these particular services. Nurses have begun to take on new technical procedures such as cryosurgery, laparoscopy and endoscopy (School of Health and Related Research 1997), and as technology develops there will be further blurring of the boundaries between medicine, nursing and HCPs (Murray et al 1995). These developments may eventually necessitate changes in the pre- and post-registration education and perhaps even regulation of all the health professional groups.

Developments in surgical procedures and the devices used in surgery have meant that many interventions now take place outside traditional surgical departments, namely in radiology units, endoscopy suites and accident and emergency departments (Vincent 1997). Consequently, work that would traditionally have been carried out by surgical nurses is now being undertaken by X-ray department nurses, clinical nurse specialists and in some instances radiographers. Some techniques, which in the past required inpatient surgical stays, are even being performed in GP surgeries. Once again this has implications for the role of practice nurses who may be required to assist.

Miller (1997) suggests that the expansion in day case surgery has also had profound effects on community health services who increasingly have to deal with post-operative conditions as well as their traditional case loads. In response to these changes, some Trusts have developed new types of service that will support patients post-operatively in the community, such as hospital-at-home schemes, but increasingly it falls to primary care workers and families to care for these patients.

Reduced length of stay

Dramatic reductions in length of hospital stay have occurred over the last decade. Between 1979 and 1990 the average length of hospital stay for patients aged 45–64 fell from just over 10 days to almost 7 days. In part, the pressure has been economic, developing from a desire to increase financial efficiency by increasing throughput. Patients are spending less time in hospital but often require more intensive input from clinicians. Developments in surgical techniques, advances in health-care knowledge and changes in philosophies regarding rehabilitation have also contributed greatly to these reductions.

Such trends have raised searching questions about the nature of health care in acute settings and in particular which clinician should provide the care. Often a new professional role has been created as a means of delivering care in ways that cross traditional professional and service boundaries. For example, new domiciliary services to support patients at home have been developed. Some Trusts have established fast-track services for cardiac patients who are discharged on day 5 post-operatively and are then visited at home by outreach cardiac home care nurses who monitor the patient's progress. In some instances the nurses have laptop computers which enable them to transmit an ECG via a modem to the patient's consultant who can then order changes in prescriptions which can be transmitted back to the nurse in the patient's home. There are also examples of other professions developing new roles in response to changes in the way services are delivered. Occupational Therapists have developed rapid discharge programmes in response to the pressure to reduce lengths of stay and have also established posts in accident and emergency departments in order to cut down inappropriate admissions to hospital.

These examples illustrate how developments in medicine and technology have radically altered the way services are delivered, which in turn impacts on the function of each of the health-care professions and the knowledge base required for practice. This is set to continue. Warner & Riley (1994) argue that developments in technology will increase the pressure to change within the health service. As a result, they postulate that the District General Hospital of the future will become a highly specialised unit treating only patients with acute needs, emergency cases and surgical day cases. Patients requiring long-term medical or rehabilitative care will be looked after in community hospitals or at home. Ranade (1997) suggests that future technological developments will open up a bewildering scenario of choice in terms of how services can be provided. Nurses and HCPs will need to be able to evaluate these choices within their own professional frameworks to ensure that services are developed in an appropriate manner.

In this chapter, so far, attempts have been made to illustrate how social policy interacts with and shapes the health professions. An underlying theme has been the impact on the health professions of key pieces of legislation and policy initiatives which have resulted in new professional roles and subsequent debates about the nature of specialist and advanced nursing and HCP practice. I now examine these developments in more detail and investigate their implications.

Medical dominance or a challenge to the traditional medical hegemony?

Annandale suggests that the most significant health-care trend in the new century will be the erasure of traditional clinical boundaries between nursing and medicine (Annandale 1998). In her analysis, which is applicable to HCPs as well as nursing, she argues that the stimulus for the shifting and blurring of professional boundaries comes from three structural factors. First, other professionals can provide some services at a lower cost and, as I have demonstrated, this factor has been important in the creation of many new health-care roles. Second, as we have seen, the reduction in junior doctors' hours of work has given nurses and HCPs the opportunity to take on new roles. Finally, Annandale suggests that nursing's own professionalisation strategy has increased the autonomy of the profession, further enabling nurses to accept new roles. But how can these shifts be interpreted? What do they mean for the long-term future of the professions?

It is interesting to ponder whether or not the developments discussed in this chapter are challenging the traditional dominance of medicine in health care or whether they merely represent a response to the continuing dominance of medicine. Walby & Greenwell (1994) suggest an analysis of the relationship between medicine and nursing which focuses on professional self interest is rather simplistic. They suggest that the changes in the relationships between medicine and nursing, including the development of new roles, can be interpreted as evidence of what has been called a 'post-Fordist' model of management in which the patient as consumer is at the centre of the service. Patterns of professional work may change and new roles develop because labour/human resources are viewed as being central to the well-running of the NHS. Clinical work is organised to enable nurses and doctors to exercise the full range of their skills and knowledge to the advantage of the patient rather than remaining in their professionally bounded spheres of responsibility. Hence new professional roles emerge that enable care to be provided in a more effective manner. If one accepts that changes in modes of delivery of health care and the emergence of new roles are not reflections of the struggles between medicine and nursing one can begin to see a subtler transfer of power within the medical profession itself, from the acute to primary sector which may indeed reflect the 'Post Fordist' model.

It is quite evident that GPs are now able to control the work of other professions including, to some extent, their professional colleagues working in Trusts. It could be argued that GPs are exercising greater control through their role as purchasers of health care and that they, as consumers, are putting the patient at the heart of the service. They are enjoying what Annandale calls 'economic leverage' in that they are able to determine not only what services, but also where services are provided (Annandale 1998). The power of GPs is likely to increase with the establishment of PCGs and as a result of the increasing emphasis on primary care. As a consequence we may see yet more changes in the way services are provided.

Liberation or subordination?

The UKCC's document, 'The scope of professional practice', has been pivotal in enabling the emergence of new nursing roles. Many commentators have argued that 'Scope' represented a culmination of the profession's maturity by allowing nurses the autonomy to determine the scope of their practice, but it could also be interpreted as a means of enabling the resubordination of nursing (Cameron & Masterson 2000). 'Scope' was launched within months of the Government's announcement of its plans to reduce the hours of work of junior doctors. As a result many commentators have argued that 'Scope' has been used to justify and promote the development of new roles that supported the needs of medicine and management rather than the needs of patients and nursing development (Dimond 1995, Denner 1995). But is this a valid interpretation of events? There is no doubt that 'Scope', the 'Junior doctors' initiative' and the development of new nursing roles will be firmly linked in popular conception partly because the research agenda at that time was focused on the need to reduce the hours of work of junior doctors. However is this hard evidence of medicine's and management's fortuitous hijacking of nursing's professional advancement or simply an example of serendipity within the world of policy formation and implementation? Is it cause and effect or coincidence?

Many of the service developments and new roles discussed in this chapter would not have been possible without a flexible, adaptable workforce, eager to develop its professional practice. It wasn't the need to reduce the hours of work of junior doctors alone that brought these developments. Waiting lists could not have been reduced without nurses and HCPs who already had the capacity to work in innovative roles. It is doubtful whether the dramatic increase in day surgery could have been achieved without a reconfiguration of traditional working patterns. At the same time technological developments have helped nurses and HCPs to perform, rather than support, many diagnostic procedures. However, perhaps this increasing flexibility shown by nursing and other health professions simply mirrors the drive for greater flexibility to be found across many employment sectors.

If we turn our attention to the wider labour market we can see that the experiences of health-care professionals reflect the experiences of those working in the computing and engineering sectors who are also having to embrace greater flexibility. Walby suggests that one of the common themes of a 'post-Fordist' reconstruction of the labour force is the creation of a layer of job-enriched functionally flexible workers. The important question is whether all workers are skilled up or whether there is a simultaneous creation of a buffer stock of poorly paid contract workers to carry out peripheral tasks (Walby & Greenwell 1994). This is a serious issue that nursing and health-care professions have to think through. Are these professions happy to countenance the development of a group of core workers who are rewarded for their greater flexibility with longer contracts, training opportunities and new titles at the expense of making a peripheral group of less qualified staff suffer insecure contracts and even lower remuneration for carrying out simpler tasks?

Conclusion

As this chapter has demonstrated, many factors have led to the creation of new professional roles. These factors have encouraged not only the blurring of professional boundaries, but have led to developments in advanced and specialist nursing and HCP practice and, quite often, to the development of new clinical roles. It has been shown how new nursing and HCP roles have developed in response to changes from within the profession and as a result of external forces.

The pace of change will almost certainly increase. As a result distinctions between health professionals and between their fields of activity will continue to blur. SNMAC (1996) argues that when new posts are conceived they should be assessed to determine whether the skills and knowledge needed to perform the role are those of a nurse. It might well be that a different profession could perform the role to better effect. As the UK health-care system develops, all the health professions must keep pace and respond to the changing demands made on them. Nurses and HCPs will need to identify and assess the drivers for change to ensure that practice develops in an appropriate manner that ensures effective patient care. 'New' does not necessarily mean 'better' and change for the sake of change should be avoided.

Witz (1994) suggested that the critical factors that would shape nursing (and arguably all of the health professions) in the 1990s would be the organisational and political contexts in which they are located and clearly that has been so. Rafferty has suggested that workforce planning in nursing has always been characterised by a combination of expediency and crisis management (Rafferty 1998). This can not continue. The challenge facing the health professions is the need to plan for the future, but even planning proactive developments can be difficult when external factors such as policy changes call for instant responses and swift action. The health professions must work in concert and ensure mutual respect.

The development of new clinical roles raises countless professional issues that will be discussed further in the following chapters. The health professions need to consider how new roles are integrated within the professional structures of the organisations in which they are based to ensure sound management. Postholders need suitable training and to have their competency assessed. Perhaps the most critical challenge is the need to balance the tension between the ever-present task of finding workforce solutions to immediate and pressing service problems and the simultaneous creation of new professional roles in a coherent manner.

REFERENCES

Annandale E (1998) The sociology of health and medicine. Polity Press, Cambridge

Audit Commission (1997) Anaesthesia under examination. HMSO, London

Baker C (1996) The health care policy process. Sage, London

Cameron A, Masterson A (2000) Social policy and nursing. In Manley K and Bellman L (eds) Surgical nursing. Churchill Livingstone, Edinburgh

Castledine G (1994) Specialist and advanced nursing and the scope of practice. In Hunt G and Wainwright P (eds) Expanding the role of the nurse. Blackwell Science, Oxford

Denner S (1995) Extending professional practice: benefits and pitfalls. Nursing Times 91(14):27–29

Department of Health (DoH) (1990) NHS and Community Care Act. HMSO, London

Department of Health (DoH) (1991a) Hours of work of doctors in training the New Deal. Executive Letter (91)82, London

Department of Health (DoH) (1991b) The patient's charter. HMSO, London

Department of Health (DoH) (1993a) Changing childbirth. Report of the Expert Maternity Group. HMSO, London

Department of Health (DoH) (1993b) Hospital doctors: training for the future. Report of the Working Group on Specialist Medical Training. Department of Health, London (Chair Sir K Calman)

Department of Health (DoH) (1997) The new NHS: modern, dependable. Stationery Office, London

Department of Health and Social Security (DHSS) (1977) The extending role of the clinical nurse – legal implications and training requirements. DHSS, London

Dimond B (1995) UKCC's standards for incorporation into contracts. British Journal of Nursing 4(18):1045–1046

Dowling S, Martin R, Skidmore P et al (1996) Nurses taking on junior doctors' work: a confusion of accountability. British Medical Journal 312:1211–1214

Doyal L, Dowling S, Cameron A (1998) Challenging practice: an evaluation of four innovatory nursing posts in the South West. Policy Press, Bristol

English T (1997) Personal paper: Medicine in the 1990s needs a team approach. British Medical Journal 314:661–663

Gough P, Maslin-Prothero S, Masterson A (1994) Nursing and social policy: care in context. Butterworth-Heinemann, Oxford

Ham C (1992) Health policy in Britain: the politics and organisation of the National Health Service, 3rd edn. Macmillan, Basingstoke

Ham C, Smith J, Temple J (1997) Hubs, spokes and policy cycles. King's Fund, London

Humphris D (1999) A framework to evaluate the role of nurse specialists. Professional Nurse 14(6):377–379

Land L, Mhaolrunaigh M A, Castledine G (1996) Extent and effectiveness of the Scope of Professional Practice. Nursing Times 96(35):32–35

Miller B (1997) Home economics. Nursing Times 93(38):32–33

Moore S (1998) Cutting edge. Guardian, 1 July

Murray C, Read S, McCabe C (1995) Reduction in junior doctors' hours: the nursing contribution. School of Health and Related Research (SCHARR), University of Sheffield, Sheffield

Nettleton S (1997) Health policy. In Ellison N, Pierson C (eds) Developments in British social policy. Macmillan, London

NHS Executive (1997) (BN NO:29/97) Improving NHS waiting lists and waiting times

NHS Management Executive (1991) Junior doctors: the New Deal. NHSME, London

Ong B N (1997) Patients approve of pre-operative assessments. Nursing Times 93(40):57–59

Paniagua H (1995) The scope of advanced practice: action potential for practice nurses. British Journal of Nursing 4(5): 269–274

Rafferty A (1998) Blurred vision. Guardian, 1 July

Ranade W (1997) A future for the NHS. Longman, London

Redfern S (1997) Reactions to nurses expanding practice. Nursing Times 93(32):45–47

Roberts-Davies M, Read S, Gilbert P, Nolan M (1998) Preparing the nurse practitioner for the 21st century. School of Nursing and Midwifery, Sheffield University

Salvage J, Wright S (1995) Nursing development units: a force for change. Scutari, London

School of Health and Related Research (SCHARR) (1997) The ENRiP data base. SCHARR, University of Sheffield, Sheffield

Standing Nursing and Midwifery Advisory Committee (SNMAC) (1996) Report of the Standing Nursing and Midwifery Advisory Committee

Tuthill V (1995) The training of nurse surgical assistants. Surgical Nurse 4(21):1240–1245

United Kingdom Central Council for Nursing, Midwifery and Health Visiting (UKCC) (1986) Project 2000: a new preparation for practice. UKCC, London

United Kingdom Central Council for Nursing, Midwifery and Health Visiting (UKCC) (1992a) The scope of professional practice. UKCC, London

United Kingdom Central Council for Nursing, Midwifery and Health Visiting (UKCC) (1992b) Code of professional conduct. UKCC, London

United Kingdom Central Council for Nursing, Midwifery and Health Visiting (UKCC) (1994) The future of professional practice – the Council's standards for education and practice following registration. UKCC, London

United Kingdom Central Council for Nursing, Midwifery and Health Visiting (UKCC) (1997) Scope in practice. UKCC, London

United Kingdom Central Council for Nursing, Midwifery and Health Visiting (UKCC) (1998) Higher level practice: papers presented to Council June 1998. UKCC, London

Vincent S (1997) The changing role of peri-operative nursing. Nursing Times 93(40):56–57

Walby S, Greenwell J (1994) Medicine and nursing: professions in a changing health service. Sage, London

Warner M, Riley C (1994) Closer to home: healthcare in the 21st century. National Association of Health Authorities and Trusts (NAHAT) Birmingham

Witz A (1994) The challenge of nursing. In Gabe J et al (eds) Challenging medicine. Routledge, London

2

The changing face of primary care
Community pharmacy

Nicola Davey

Introduction

In this chapter the changing face of primary care is considered from the perspective of the community pharmacist. The way in which pharmacists' roles have changed over time is explored in relation to issues within and external to the profession, both in the past and now in response to the formation of Primary Care Groups and Primary Care Trusts (Department of Health 1997).

Pharmacy has the potential to become a leading provider of health care. Utilising their vast expertise on the effective use of medicines and their position in the high street, pharmacists offer services which range from supporting self-care and responding to the symptoms of self-limiting illness to chronic disease management. They are also valuable information resources to support those involved in using medicines, from selecting, prescribing, supplying and administering them, through to advising on adverse effects, side-effects and contraindications, and optimum use. This chapter touches upon some of the fundamental factors that will determine whether their potential will be fully realised or if pharmacists will remain tied to the dispensing bench for ever.

In this first section the history of community pharmacy is examined through key elements that define the individual and the service: the profession's origin; the supervision requirement; service configuration; qualifications; skill mix; multiprofessional contact; remuneration packages; and the 1990 reforms. In the second section the roles of professional organisations are examined briefly in relation to regulation, advisory functions, training, and negotiation on behalf of individuals, independent contractors and multiples. Drawing on the literature in the third section, models of practice are examined and discussed in light of the changing roles of pharmacists and other caring professions. Finally in the fourth section the new opportunities and challenges for community pharmacy are considered, starting with the short term and then looking forward to the challenges that will need to be faced in the long term, in particular the pressure to control escalating public expenditure on drugs and meeting demands from a more informed population.

A brief history of community pharmacy

Today there are over 22 000 pharmacists practising in approximately 12 500 community pharmacies throughout the UK, but the evolution from apothecary to pharmacist has been slow. In this section the position of pharmacy or the high-street chemist is compared to general practice. Charting the profession's origin, the supervision requirement and changes in service configuration, level of qualifications, skill mix and multiprofessional working, the constraints of the existing remuneration framework are apparent. This historical perspective takes us up to and includes developments that have occurred as a result of the 1990 reforms (Department of Health 1989). Although pharmacy is small when compared with other health professions a number of the elements discussed here will have a familiar ring to them.

Until the formation of the NHS many people's experience of primary care consisted of an infrequent visit to a doctor working alone from a surgery in the GP's own home. Primary care has come a long way since 1948, and whilst some GPs still practise alone many are in partnership with other GPs, employ practice nurses, and work from health centres or purpose-built premises.

Investment in health centres by health authorities from the 1960s enabled a more diverse group of health-care professionals to practise from the same location. On rare occasions pharmacies were incorporated into the new premises or located adjacent to them, offering the chance of greater contact between the health-care professions. However, the majority of community pharmacies have remained highly accessible to the public in prime high-street sites, but strangely isolated from the rest of the primary care team.

The rise of GP fundholding in the 1990s offered some GPs the opportunity to bring together a more diverse range of primary care practitioners under one roof, thus extending the core primary care team. On occasion this included pharmacists who provided prescribing advice and even medicines management clinics within the surgery, although this was down to individual persistence on the part of pharmacists rather than any national recognition of their collective skills.

Like general practice, community pharmacy in 1948 comprised mainly independent contractors. Most commonly practising from high-street premises, they would traditionally have been supported by one or two shop assistants. Unlike in some parts of Europe, UK legislation did not require or restrict pharmacists to the role of sole proprietor but did require pharmacists to supervise dispensing and over-the-counter sales of medicines at all times. In 1999 large national and multinational pharmacy chains comprised 32% of pharmacies in the UK, and small groups of pharmacies comprised 40%, the rest being independents. Most large stores will employ at least two pharmacists, one to manage the store and one to supervise the dispensary, allowing some flexibility. This may be an important factor in the future since the statutory supervision requirement means that one pharmacist must always be available to oversee all dispensing and medicine sales.

The configuration of community pharmacy in the 1990s is to a large extent a legacy from the 1970s and 1980s, when the absence of restrictions on new pharmacies fuelled a rapid explosion in numbers and consequently a demand for pharmacists. This situation prevailed until an amendment to the regulations in 1987 required new applicants for contracts to demonstrate that this was necessary or desirable for a locality. Current requirements can be found in the 'National Health Service (Pharmaceutical Services) Regulations 1992 SI no. 662'. Community pharmacy has therefore moved from a service exclusively composed of independent contractors to one strongly influenced by multiple chains. This also means that pharmacists now have a choice of employment status ranging from sole owner, to employee as a dispensary or store manager through to professional locum.

The pharmacy qualification has also evolved from a vocational training to a 3-year degree course (4 years in Scotland), with a 1-year compulsory vocational training. From 2000 this will increase to a 4-year degree course (in England and Wales), creating a fallow year in which no graduates will become pre-registration students. This short-term workforce crisis will coincide with a much more serious chronic shortage of practising community and hospital pharmacists throughout England and Wales.

As with many other health professions, time pressures on pharmacists have placed greater emphasis on the role of support staff. In community pharmacy the trained dispenser has become a vital link, whilst the broader remit of the pharmacy technician through a National Vocational Qualification confers additional skills in manufacturing and some aspects of therapeutics. Following high-profile media criticism of pharmacy counter assistants in the early 1990s, protocols were introduced to guide the sales of over-the-counter medicines in 1995. In 1996 a requirement was introduced for anyone involved in the sale of medicines to have completed a relevant accredited training course. Increasing skill mix amongst community pharmacy support staff has enabled a gradual change in the pharmacist's role. From the public's point of view this is perhaps most notable in the increased visibility of pharmacists as they have moved from the back-room dispensary towards the counter.

Whilst pharmacists do not have a personal list in the same way as general practitioners, nor case loads as in the managed services, the introduction, and remuneration, of patient medication records (PMRs) is a step forward. Pharmacists now receive a small payment for keeping computerised records of prescribed medication dispensed to regular customers. However, many existing systems and records remain incomplete as they do not yet have the facility to record over-the-counter sales. Despite this limitation the PMR does allow pharmacists to take a more proactive role in providing high-quality pharmaceutical care for people who return to the same pharmacy on a regular basis. However, this would need to be developed much further for pharmacists to fulfil a pharmaceutical practitioner role as discussed later in the chapter. Other personalised services such as prescription collection and delivery are also a step forward in meeting the needs of many older people, but these have been driven by competition for business rather than any direct remuneration for the enhanced service being provided.

As in other health-care professions, a number of extended roles have been suggested and piloted by pharmacists over the last two decades. However, regardless of the protocols and procedures adopted, the supervision requirement which ties the pharmacist to the pharmacy, combined with the absence of nationally agreed remuneration packages, has prevented them from becoming core activities. With the exception of pharmacists located in health centres, these constraints have hindered the development of joint training and integration of pharmacists with the wider primary care team. Despite good working relationships within the pharmacy, recognition and awareness of the pharmacist's potential contribution amongst other members of the primary care team has generally been low.

Whilst the framework for remuneration may seem of little consequence to those working in the managed sector, it is a crucial factor in determining the ability of any independent practitioner to embrace new roles. Pharmacists receive payment from a global sum and, whilst the range of payments are simpler to understand and administer than those made to general practitioners, they are also much less wide-ranging. The current system provides a fee per item thereby rewarding pharmacists for dispensing prescriptions, rather than providing professional services. As mentioned earlier, the desire to explore extended roles for pharmacists began in the 1970s and continued throughout the 1980s and 1990s. It is therefore disappointing to find that by the end of the 1990s national guidance on remuneration for services, other than dispensing, was limited to two areas:

- Directed Pharmacy Services, covering needle exchange schemes, provision of advice to nursing and residential homes, provision of oxygen, participation in emergency duty rotas
- Professional Allowance, reflecting the service element of dispensing (and related to volume of prescriptions dispensed), the maintenance of PMRs and the display of health promotion leaflets.

Although the 1990 NHS reforms (Department of Health 1989) did bring new opportunities for a wider range of professions to provide services within the primary care setting, a lack of flexibility and movement on remuneration has done little to enhance the role of community pharmacists. Despite prescribing being consistently on the policy and economic agendas, investment and incentives have historically been oriented towards general practitioners with little recognition of the many other skills relating to medicines and medicines use practised daily by community pharmacists. Notable exceptions did occur within fundholding, where investment in adding a pharmacist to the primary care team was often found to be both cost-effective and popular (Tordoff & Wright 1999, Hughes, Turner & Fitzpatrick 1999).

The Health Authority advisory roles that accompanied these reforms tended to favour pharmacists from the managed service with a background in drug information and hospital pharmacy services. Over the decade many advisers did, against the odds, justify investment in small-scale service development to build on existing pharmacy skills with a slow but steady creation of pharmacy facilitators providing a vital link with community pharmacists. At the same time nursing advisers were, in a similar mode, developing the practice nurse role, although the nursing profession as a whole took a much longer-term view than its pharmacy counterparts.

Professional organisations

Most health-care professions are associated with several organisations offering a range of services from professional registration, regulation and monitoring, to negotiation, education, training and professional development. The range of organisations that exists for any profession reflects its evolution, development and, perhaps most importantly, the demands of the environment in which its members practise. With the 1998 reforms it is likely that clinical governance will be added to the areas covered (Department of Health 1997). All major health professions have a professional body with responsibility for registration, maintaining professional standards and protecting the public. In some cases this is their sole remit: for example, the United Kingdom Central Council for Nursing, Midwifery and Health Visiting. In pharmacy the Royal Pharmaceutical Society of Great Britain (RPSGB) undertakes registration. It also covers professional standards, education, professional development, clinical audit, law and ethics, practice research and the development of pharmaceutical sciences. Through its membership services it provides a network of local branches offering an informal opportunity for pharmacists to meet socially, hear presentations and debate professional matters. Every year it hosts an annual conference for all parts of the profession.

Whilst the RPSGB supports continuing professional development as good professional practice, it is not yet obligatory. Movements to encourage pharmacists to take personal responsibility for their personal learning portfolios are some way behind professions such as nursing. Government-sponsored continuing education programmes are coordinated centrally through the Centre for Postgraduate Pharmaceutical Education and its counterparts in Wales, Scotland and Northern Ireland. Whilst they are generally of a high quality they may be less well suited to meet the demand for flexible, multi-professional learning that the new Primary Care Groups and Trusts will require, and that clinical governance will demand (Department of Health 1997).

The National Pharmaceutical Association (NPA) is a trade organisation founded originally to support the small independent pharmacy. As small local chains formed and grew, some eventually merged to become national chains maintaining their membership throughout. Consequently the NPA today has membership from most independent pharmacies, small chains, cooperatives and nationals (with the exception of Boots the Chemist). The services it offers its members range from business services; merchandising advice; personal and business insurance and professional indemnity; providing training courses for dispensing and counter assistants; drug information; and professional advice. Since 1995 the NPA has also invested in regional coordinators to share good practice and liaise between Health Authorities and pharmacists to explore local service development. The contribution that the NPA has made to developing pharmacy support staff cannot be underestimated, as it is the key to pharmacists utilising their substantial education, skills and training in the future.

The Pharmaceutical Services Negotiating Committee (PSNC) along with its counterpart in Scotland, is the profession's union, representing individual and company contractors. The central committees negotiate the global sum of money available to pharmacy each year and the way in which this is earned. The PSNC keeps in touch with its members through the Local Pharmaceutical Committees (LPCs). For many years the Committee did little to encourage its members to explore extended roles on the basis that extra remuneration was not on offer. However, in the last few years there has been more cooperation between the three bodies, the PSNC, NPA and the RPSGB, in specific areas such as medicines management and premises development.

As mentioned earlier in this section, the RPSGB has an interest in the education that pharmacists receive. In the case of undergraduates this requires that their course provides the foundation on which registration is based. Practical experience is then gained in the pre-registration year. Undergraduate degree programmes will, from the year 2000, be extended from 3 to 4 years to accommodate the growing demands on the curriculum, particularly in relation to developments in primary care. With greater emphasis being placed on health economics, evidence-based health care, the application of technology and clinical audit, the aim is to support and promote good prescribing management. Coverage of social pharmacy and health promotion issues will also be increased. Although some Schools of Pharmacy are moving towards multiprofessional learning, in general pharmacy has been slow to embrace what some might see as an obvious, necessary and long-overdue progression.

This structural overview touches on areas of tension that lie within the pharmacy profession, and to some extent within general and independent practice. First, there is the tension between care versus commerce; second, the rivalry between different professional organisations; and third, there is competition between individuals and companies. Whilst all these tensions can contribute to maintaining the momentum for change that is now required in health care, too little can cause inertia and too much can be destabilising. Whilst individuals and multinational companies will compete rigorously on established territory, the task of forging a new service is most often championed by a handful of entrepreneurs whose investment can only be realised if and when the system catches up with their innovation.

During the 1980s, amongst growing frustration with the protocols and inertia that often pervade remote institutions, the Young Pharmacists Group was formed, demanding room for a new voice in the profession's destiny. In the early 1990s further tensions between the professional body, its modus operandi and the membership became apparent, leading ultimately to a bold stock-take on an unprecedented scale.

The launch of a discussion paper in 1995 entitled 'Pharmacy in a new age' developed a strategy for the future of pharmacy (Royal Pharmaceutical Society of Great Britain 1995) and marked a radical new approach for the Society. Reflecting many similar debates raised by nursing in the 'Heathrow' debate (Department of Health 1994), it attempted to bridge the chasm between the institution and the individual. Using a series of thought-provoking bulletins, a consultation process was begun with the membership, and the 5000 responses were honed down to an agenda for action containing 22 items. From this work 'Building the future', the future strategy for pharmaceutical services, was launched (Royal Pharmaceutical Society of Great Britain 1996). The consultation process to this point had involved a significant proportion of the profession, lasted 2 years, and finally identified five key areas central to future pharmacy practice, together with a series of supporting aims. These areas covered:

◆ management of prescribed medicines
◆ management of long-term conditions
◆ management of common ailments
◆ promotion and support of healthy lifestyles
◆ advice and support for other health-care professionals.

The key supporting aims included: information; education and training; evidence-based practice; standards of practice; workforce remuneration; distribution of community pharmacies; improvement of premises; and commitment to progress. Clinical governance and audit would probably feature explicitly if the aims were to be reviewed today.

To address the challenge of translating the strategy into recognised patterns of practice a series of road shows were undertaken and the formation of a network of coordinators, led to the setting up of local pharmacy development groups across the UK. Letting go from the centre is never easy; motivating people from a variety of local pharmacy organisations, with different agendas, to meet together and support strategically focused developments is a significant challenge. Yet a much larger challenge is still to come, in returning this agenda to those who originally shaped it, individual practising pharmacists, and in ensuring the chasm between institution and member never becomes so great again.

Models of practice and emerging roles

In the early 1990s Hepler & Strand (1990) described the evolution of the pharmacy profession, analysing changes in the role which occurred as a response to the major economic shifts from the agricultural through the industrial to the information eras. The pharmacist moved from a compounding function in the early part of this century (mixtures, potions and lotions) towards a predominantly supply function (dispensing tablets and capsules). During the last two decades the supply function was rejected in favour of one that recognised and utilised the pharmacist's scientific and medical training; this is known as early clinical pharmacy (advising on safety, appropriateness and cost-effectiveness of drugs). In the 1990s a further development emerged to reflect the shift towards the social welfare function of pharmacists, a

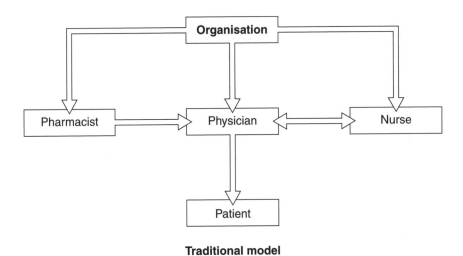

Traditional model

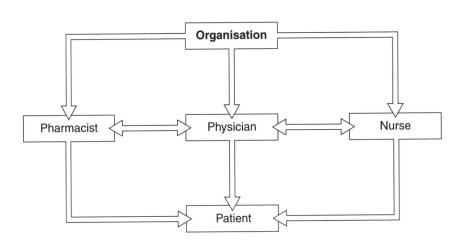

Practitioner model

Figure 2.1 Indirect and direct practitioner–patient relationships

concept which has been described as pharmaceutical care. This approach places a greater emphasis on the pharmaceutical practitioner's responsibilities towards, and relationships with, patients rather than organisations or other professions as a first line of care (Fig. 2.1).

The importance of pharmacists understanding the different responsibilities they have towards their patients, colleagues and organisations is fundamental to this evolutionary process, but has parallels with other professions. All non-medical professions wishing to establish a new role must determine when, and how, their obligations to the patient take precedence over obligations to others. Compared with the more traditional model which places pharmacists, nurses and other health-care professions in support of a doctor, the practitioner model can establish explicitly the direct relationship with the patient (see Fig. 2.1). Whilst this might seem straightforward, the implicit expectations and historical balance of power suggest that such a transition is extremely complex and requires significant investment to effect a long-term cultural shift (Fig. 2.2).

Although various definitions have been put forward for pharmaceutical care, most recently Cippole et al (1998) have proposed the following: 'A practice in which the practitioner takes responsibility for a patient's drug-related needs and is held accountable for this commitment'. However, they concluded that no single profession is capable of providing quality care in isolation from others and suggested that care systems need to support cooperation between a number of professions as well as the patient to achieve positive patient outcomes. Since 1990, Cippole et al (1998) have developed and tested

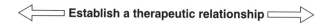

Establish a therapeutic relationship

Assessment	Care Planning	Evaluation
• Ensure all drug therapy is indicated, effective, safe and convenient • Identify drug therapy problems to resolve and prevent	• Resolve drug therapy problems • Achieve therapeutic goals • Prevent drug therapy problems	• Record actual patient outcomes • Evaluate progress in meeting therapeutic goals • Reassess for new problems

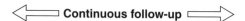

Continuous follow-up

Figure 2.2 Model of pharmaceutical care, Cippole, Strand & Morley (1998)

a pharmaceutical model in Minnesota, USA. The three core elements of pharmaceutical care and some of the subprocesses shown in Figure 2.2 may be familiar to other professions including nurses. However, significant long-term investment is required at many levels of the pharmacy profession to develop the detail needed for practitioners to take responsibility for meeting all drug-related needs. They have also explored the pharmacist's role in relationship to the patient/client and other health-care professions using a wheel to illustrate different elements of professional care together with the patient's own self-care, as shown in Figure 2.3.

In the UK pharmaceutical care has been discussed for over a decade, and in 1992 a joint working party considered the future role of the community pharmaceutical services. They produced a report on behalf of the Department of Health and the pharmaceutical profession, 'Pharmaceutical Care: the future for community pharmacy' (Royal Pharmaceutical Society of Great Britain 1992). The group produced 30 recommendations, several of which would provide the foundations on which pharmaceutical care could evolve and perhaps flourish. However, many of the recommendations have yet to leave the drawing board and a UK model of pharmaceutical care and the commitment to invest in a sustainable infrastructure have yet to emerge.

Instead, medicines review and medicines management pilot programmes have begun to flourish. Whilst there is great scope for improved quality of care and greater cost-effectiveness as a result of medicines review, responsibility

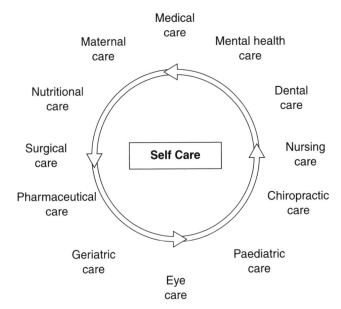

Figure 2.3 Health-care needs of a patient, Cippole, Strand & Morley (1998)

for the patient's care remains firmly with the general practitioner, and indeed the pharmacist working in a surgery may never see the patient. The pharmacist makes recommendations that may be accepted or rejected. Medicines management, on the other hand, will often combine the prescription review with patient contact, enabling the pharmacist to interact and establish specific care issues including the patient's attitudes and beliefs about his or her medicines. However, the relationship between the pharmacist and the patient remains indirect, with the GP taking responsibility for the medicines ultimately provided.

Although there is support for the concept of pharmaceutical care across the United Kingdom, to date little funding has been committed and it is in Scotland where the first attempt has been made to adapt the American model and demonstrate its use within a framework for community-based NHS pharmacy services, as shown in Figure 2.4 (Clinical Resource and Audit Group 1999).

Although needs assessment relating to individual patients, rather than population needs, is now an integral part of social services and other health-care professions, it is not yet formally recognised as a core pharmacy activity, despite being an implicit part of most pharmacists' daily work. However, for pharmacists to identify patient-focused care issues within the pharmaceutical care plan they must consider the very different types of goal and expectation that might be sought. In this respect they must be able to separate the practitioner expression of need from the patient expression of need by giving

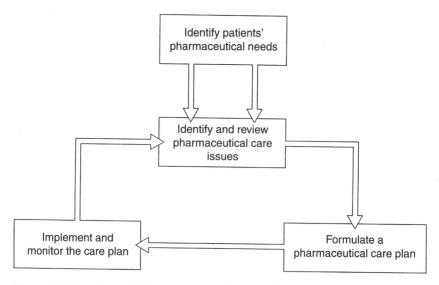

Figure 2.4 Scottish model for pharmaceutical care

equal weighting to the patient's expectation of medicines, encompassing their beliefs and lifestyle issues. The term 'concordance' has been attributed to this approach.

As a result of a consultation begun in 1995, 'From compliance to concordance – achieving shared goals in medicine' was published in 1997 (Royal Pharmaceutical Society of Great Britain 1997). Supported by an extensive literature review, a group representing medicine, psychology, pharmacy and nursing promoted the use of the term 'concordance' to encompass a broader meaning than the more traditional terms 'adherence' and 'compliance'. The concept assumes a negotiation between equals, i.e. that a therapeutic alliance is created between the prescriber and the patient which may ultimately include an agreement to differ. Whilst this work related specifically to the use of medicines there are many situations pertaining to people with chronic conditions where the concept can be applied to other aspects of care. This is in keeping with a desire by some to empower individuals to participate more actively in decisions regarding their health. The pharmaceutical practitioner model and concordance are two major concepts that may determine the destiny of the pharmacy profession in the 21st century. The five areas outlined in the consultation process set out a framework within which the profession will be defined. In the next section we look at some of the new opportunities that are arising in response to the 1997 reforms (Department of Health 1997) and consider the short- and long-term implications for the profession.

Realising opportunities in primary care

The Government's reforms of the NHS across the UK represent the most significant development in primary care for almost a decade. In England the introduction of a whole new framework including Health Improvement Programmes (HImPs), the Commission for Health Improvement (CHI), the National Institute for Clinical Excellence (NICE) and clinical governance, together with changing skill mix and the blurring of boundaries with social care will be major policy drivers influencing all health practice in the longer term. However, before we consider the long-term implications for community pharmacy practice let us examine the short-term implications of the reforms.

Short-term implications

The formation of Primary Care Groups (PCGs) and subsequently Primary Care Trusts (PCTs) follows a path already familiar to hospitals and fundholding practices, the key difference being the inclusive, rather than the exclusive, nature of membership and the drive towards cooperative rather than competitive arrangements. The speed of the formation of PCGs, Primary Care Commissioning Pilots in Northern Ireland (Department of Health and Social Services Northern Ireland 1999), Local Health Care Cooperatives in Scotland (The Scottish Office 1997) and Local Health Groups in Wales (The Welsh Office 1998) is both unprecedented and challenging, with many operational groups emerging less than a year from their announcement.

The stream of government publications and initiatives that were issued during Labour's first year in power were presented as informing a 10-year plan but the rate of implementation has been overwhelming. Any profession waiting for tasks or services to appear with their names attached will have been disappointed. As the various parts of the NHS responded, it became clear that each profession would need to identify its own particular contribution and be proactive in establishing links with others. For many professions a swift stock-take and quick manœuvring were needed to grasp new opportunities.

The introduction of cash-limited prescribing for the whole of primary care represented a powerful driver for change unleashed in 1999 on (with the exception of fundholding GPs) a largely unsuspecting audience within primary care. Significant changes in any funding stream will always hasten responses, but the magnitude of the prescribing budget as a proportion of total primary care spend makes this change worthy of note. With prescribing costs representing approximately 13% of all NHS costs (over £4.5 billion in 1999) and up to 20% of PCT budgets, the shift of prescribing costs from a non-cash-limited amount to a global cash-limited sum is significant. Demand for people with the skills to analyse prescribing costs and trends combined with the skills to influence prescribing at both strategic and practice levels was unprecedented. The challenge was to find such people in the absence of a nationally defined infrastructure and strategic development programme.

Earlier in this chapter the effect of an inflexible remuneration structure on development of pharmacy services was considered, with the net result being a proliferation of projects that were by necessity small-scale, local and diverse. Despite this, over a period of 10 years a slow revolution has occurred with small numbers of community pharmacists gaining limited experience of working with GPs on aspects of prescribing ranging from repeat prescribing to drug formulary projects. When the opportunity arose it was therefore this group of pharmacists that formed the first wave of prescribing support pharmacists working in PCGs and in general practice across the country. Working within terms and conditions determined outside of the national community pharmacy remuneration framework, this situation provides yet another example of the failure to develop a modern infrastructure that can accommodate evolving pharmacy practice.

In the short term, therefore, an opportunity has been created for a proportion of community pharmacists to move forward in a new direction, utilising many previously underused skills, a situation that perhaps echoes the position of nurse specialists a decade ago. However, a number of issues rooted in the pharmacy profession's history remain to be overcome, not least of which is the need for a flexible remuneration structure if this new role is to be consolidated in the medium to long term. Whilst pharmacists and companies can invest in the provision of such services outside of the contract, Health Authorities and PCGs are unable to realign the global sum currently available to pharmacists to support this. Instead they must find new money for pharmacists, from other sources. Whilst the prescribing budget is currently a popular source, it brings with it a different set of limitations on the development of any new role.

Ideally investment is required to develop remunerated pharmacy-based support services that complement practice-based services. If a fragmented approach is to be avoided, greater investment will be required in the infrastructure to support pharmacist development both within and outside of their traditional working environment, and models of pharmaceutical care need to be tested and evaluated to develop appropriate and sustainable models of service delivery.

The obstacles to overcoming the shortage of pharmacists and enabling them to have more scope to develop new roles within primary care could be conquered. Two solutions have been hotly debated but the issue has never been resolved within the profession. The first is to reduce the number of pharmacies, enabling more pharmacists to cover each premises; the second is to increase skill mix and level of qualification amongst pharmacy staff whilst introducing an amendment to the supervision requirement, thus allowing some flexibility for pharmacists to leave the premises. It remains to be seen how long this important issue will remain unresolved.

For pharmacy and other health and social care professions there are important lessons to be learnt from the significant changes in funding streams. Whilst greater flexibility across primary and secondary care and even social care boundaries may arise as a result of the 1998 reforms, it is also clear that much of this flexibility may be countered or curtailed by the 'labelling' of new funding streams to meet specific strategic objectives. The introduction of the modernisation fund, for example, included money for computerisation and nursing pay awards amongst other things, and the use of waiting list initiative money has for some time been centrally directed.

In light of the above, chief executives and PCG and PCT boards and managers cannot fail to realise the immense challenge that managing prescribing represents. Whilst in the short term there are still financial savings to be made, a much greater challenge is presented. Pharmacy and the skills that pharmacists have need to be valued in the bigger picture if quality of life is to be improved through the effective use of drugs, whether directly by those providing pharmaceutical care or indirectly through support for prescribers. The demand for the skills of pharmacists has never been more apparent, nor the challenge greater, but their development agenda needs to be seen in the context of the environment that is being created in the longer term.

Longer-term implications

In the longer term PCGs and PCTs will need to deliver services within National Service Frameworks and develop services in the broader context of the Health Improvement Programme (HImP). New drugs and technologies will be used within guidance provided by the National Institute for Clinical Excellence (NICE) and clinical governance will drive changes in clinical practice. As if this agenda is not sufficiently challenging, at the same time a number of key changes to service delivery are being introduced, including Primary Care Trusts, NHS Direct, and Walk-in clinics. Although these will have an immediate effect within the primary care sector, their impact is likely to be felt in secondary care and social care as well.

NHS Direct and Walk-in clinics are regarded on the one hand with optimism and on the other with suspicion. Whilst there are undoubtedly considerable problems that need to be resolved at the interface with traditional primary care, there is clearly a perceived public appetite for such services. Some pharmacists may well claim to provide much of what NHS Direct provides in a more personal setting, in a shorter space of time and with more direct referral to local providers; a few may already provide this service by telephone to vulnerable people. However, in this 24-hour information and service age, pharmacists will need to demonstrate and market the added value that they deliver if they are to persuade purchasers to invest in helping them overcome the barriers. On a positive note, the NPA has received funding to explore closer links between pharmacy and NHS Direct, a development that will be followed closely by those with any interest in our profession's future. Whilst many GPs perceive walk-in clinics as a threat to general practice, Boots the Chemist in Birmingham is host to one of the first pilot NHS walk-in centres. Building on a model that is already familiar to a small number of multiples and independent pharmacies across the country, the new walk-in services will also have links with NHS Direct, local GPs, hospitals, social services and voluntary services. The range of influences in the environment that will shape these changes is set out in Figure 2.5.

Reflecting national and local priorities, the HImP will increasingly focus resources on issues that represent major causes of morbidity and mortality, with coronary heart disease, cancer and mental health likely to feature for the foreseeable future. Coordinated by the Health Authority, the HImP will

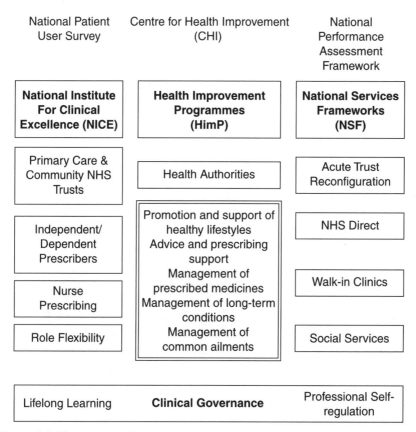

National Patient User Survey

Centre for Health Improvement (CHI)

National Performance Assessment Framework

National Institute For Clinical Excellence (NICE)

Health Improvement Programmes (HimP)

National Services Frameworks (NSF)

Primary Care & Community NHS Trusts

Health Authorities

Acute Trust Reconfiguration

Independent/ Dependent Prescribers

Promotion and support of healthy lifestyles
Advice and prescribing support
Management of prescribed medicines
Management of long-term conditions
Management of common ailments

NHS Direct

Nurse Prescribing

Walk-in Clinics

Role Flexibility

Social Services

Lifelong Learning

Clinical Governance

Professional Self-regulation

Figure 2.5 The range of influences shaping pharmacy practice

provide a longer-term strategy for all local initiatives and these will increasingly be combined to form a joint strategy with social care. There will be strong pressure for funding streams to be aligned with the HImP although other national priorities may emerge as a result of work undertaken by the Standing Medical Advisory Committee (1998) on the use of antibiotics, and from new institutions such as NICE.

For community pharmacists the launch of the HImP comes at a time when the prevention of illness and treatment of minor illness have been recognised within the national professional strategy, along with the management of long-term conditions. The potential for pharmacists to contribute to needs assessment for people who rarely access mainstream primary care and social services could also be realised within this context. In relation to NICE, pharmacists are increasingly recognised for their ability to support an evidence-based approach to medicine, both in their interaction with the public and by providing support to other professions involved with the prescribing and administration of medicines. Using the latest information technology and given their accessibility the provision of information is one role that pharmacists should be well placed to fulfil. Once again, pharmacists in the UK have much to learn from what is available in the USA. As a profession we must be clear of the benefits and risks of direct access to medicines that the Internet may bring and be sure to offer attractive alternatives including personal and local pharmaceutical care services, particularly for those with chronic illness.

There is the potential for great advances if some of the changes to prescribing status proposed in the 'Crown report' (Department of Health 1999) are implemented. The 'Crown report' considered the use of patient group directions to cover the supply and administration of medicines, whilst the final report defined two new prescribing roles that may apply to new professional groups (i.e. non-doctors). Independent prescribers, as the name suggests, will be able to prescribe medicines from a limited list within specified therapeutic areas of care. District nurses and health visitors who have become nurse prescribers provide an example of the model of independent prescribers developed within existing legislation. Dependent prescribers will be able to initiate therapy following medical diagnosis with an expression of intention to treat and to continue or modify an original prescription on repeat. Despite considerable resistance from the medical profession for community pharmacists to be given dependent prescriber status it is quite clear that pharmacists already act as independent prescribers when they respond to symptoms and provide recommendations on over-the-counter medicines. Whilst doctors might consider this of little significance, the number of prescription drugs which have been rescheduled to over-the-counter status in the last decade provides the pharmacist with considerable scope. Although these new prescribing roles present a significant challenge to many of the health professions and require primary legislation, they recognise and legitimise the role non-doctors already play in many aspects of practice. Such legislation should establish explicit boundaries, provide a mechanism for review and recognise the need for appropriate training and support. In the long term many pharmacists and nurses may become dependent prescribers and in a few cases independent prescribers, but whatever the outcome of the 'Crown report' for pharmacists, they will continue to provide support to others who achieve this status.

Changing expectations amongst the public and a desire to provide a more responsive service resulted in the launch of NHS Direct. Still in its infancy, it will take time to establish the part this and other innovations such as one-stop health clinics will play in primary care in the 21st century, although their potential success may be weakened if traditional professional boundaries continue to create limits to what is possible. There is a new opportunity for

Primary Care Trusts to embrace many more primary care professions within a managed or semi-managed service, which may ultimately lead to the redefinition, rather than demise, of the role of independent general medical practitioners (Beecham 1999).

Organisations, professions and individuals will need to be proactive if they are to master clinical governance. Organisations will need to build the infrastructure to support those who are underachieving by dealing fairly and honestly with both managerial and clinical shortcomings. Professions charged with self-regulation will need to encourage their members to respond through re-registration, commitment to lifelong learning, peer review and audit. Services will need to become more user-focused, with less emphasis on professional self-interest. Finally each professional will need to take greater responsibility for the care she or he provides, not in isolation from others but within the context of the total care that is provided.

When we look at organisational maps and diagrams showing professional relationships it is perhaps not uncommon to scan first for our own position and that of our patients or clients before looking more broadly at those around us. Looking from a pharmacy perspective we might traditionally have

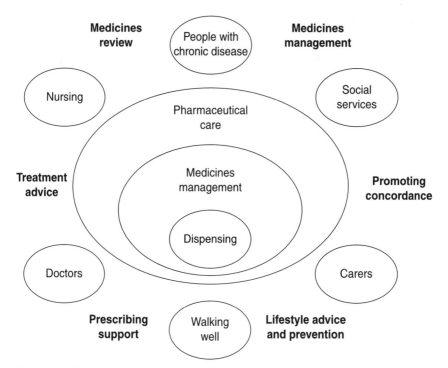

Figure 2.6 Ripple of pharmacy interactions with the public and other health-care sectors

considered the customer/patient, GP and nurse, with the hospital in the distance, but looking around at primary care now we find a much more diverse and rapidly changing picture, with a rich array of macro and micro changes in the health-care professions and related systems opening up new opportunities to use our skills. Figure 2.6 shows some of the interfaces between pharmacy and other health and care providers.

Conclusion

Pharmacy is an underutilised profession in need of greater conviction, momentum, long-term strategic planning and cooperation between stake-holders to resolve problems and provide support for its champions. One priority must be a remuneration structure that is more responsive to innovation and rewards services provided instead of putting pills in pots; another must be the ability for pharmacists to work within their pharmacies and out in their community on the same day.

Pharmacists are highly trained people whose most important contribution is the knowledge they can give to others on the appropriate, safe, cost-effective and optimum use of medicines. They are situated in prime high-street locations. They could have access to a massive range of information on drugs using the latest technology, and furthermore be able to communicate this to the public in ways that they readily understand. They can provide a social function, identifying problems and directing people to services that they need. They see the walking well and the sick, but they can't leave the premises during the day to visit a patient, join practice meetings in the local surgery or attend joint training without another pharmacist being employed or closing the pharmacy.

The pharmacists who now counsel patients on medicines use, join practice meetings in the local surgery and attend joint training often do not work in the local pharmacy. They have put together their own portfolio of work, providing prescribing support to GPs and nurses by tapping into the prescribing budget for funding. They have little job security and uncertain career pathways, but high satisfaction from using their skills in different settings and interacting with other professions. Some are already extending into medicines management and will progress towards providing pharmaceutical care. Yet it is still not apparent when, where and how pharmaceutical practitioners will become a reality.

Links are already forming between pharmacy and the new players on the block. Prescribing support will become increasingly important for PCGs as they become PCTs, and resources become ever more stretched. Pharmacists are working with NHS Direct and have a wealth of experience in the front line to bring to such a service. Walk-in clinics will not go away although their client groups may become more clearly defined, and some will be based in community pharmacies.

At the beginning of this chapter the potential for community pharmacists to become leading providers of health care was suggested. Having read this, you may now have a little more insight into the fundamental factors that will determine the outcome for pharmacy and be considering some of the similarities and differences between pharmacists, nurses and other health-care professionals. The 21st century holds many promises for pharmacy and many more for primary care as professions begin working together in a more complementary and holistic way to deliver patient-focused care. The key message for all health professions must be to learn about and respect the contributions made by others. No profession should be shy of saying what its contribution to a person's care might be in certain circumstances for fear of encroaching on another's territory, but should be ready to pass on responsibility when a professional is no longer the appropriate person to meet the patient or client's needs. Whilst there may be a blurring of professional boundaries we should be wary of becoming a jack of all trades, and instead be a master of at least one that delivers health gain.

REFERENCES

Beecham L (1999) UK GPs will produce blueprint for the future. British Medical Journal 319:12
Cippole R J, Strand L M, Morley P C (1998) Pharmaceutical care practice. McGraw-Hill, New York
Clinical Resource and Audit Group (1999) Clinical pharmacy practice in primary care. The Scottish Office, Edinburgh Stationery Office
Department of Health DoH (1989) Working for patients. HMSO, London
Department of Health DoH (1994) The challenges for nursing and midwifery in the 21st century (the Heathrow debate). HMSO, London
Department of Health DoH (1997) The new NHS: modern, dependable. Stationery Office, London
Department of Health (1999) Review of prescribing, supply and administration of medicines: final report (Chair Dame June Crown), Stationery Office, London
Department of Health and Social Services Northern Ireland (1999) Fit for the future – a new approach. DHSS NI, Belfast
Hepler C, Strand L (1990) Opportunities and responsibilities in pharmaceutical care. American Journal of Hospital Pharmacy 47:533–543
Hughes C M, Turner K, Fitzpatrick C (1999) The use of a prescribing audit tool to assess the impact of a practice pharmacist in general practice. Pharmaceutical Journal 262:27–30
Royal Pharmaceutical Society of Great Britain (1992) Pharmaceutical care: the future for community pharmacy. RPSGB, London
Royal Pharmaceutical Society of Great Britain (1995) Pharmacy in a new age – the shape of things to come. RPSGB, London
Royal Pharmaceutical Society of Great Britain (1996) Pharmacy in a new age – the new horizon. RPSGB, London
Royal Pharmaceutical Society of Great Britain (1997) From compliance to concordance – achieving shared goals in medicine. RPSGB, London

Standing Medical Advisory Committee (1998) The path of least resistance. Department of Health, London

The Scottish Office (1997) Designed to care: renewing the National Health Service in Scotland. The Scottish Office, Edinburgh Stationery Office

The Welsh Office (1998) Putting patients first. The Welsh Office, Cardiff

Tordoff J, Wright D (1999) Analysis of the impact of community pharmacists providing formulary development advice to GPs. Pharmaceutical Journal 262:166–168

3

Research, evaluation and evidence-based practice

Sarah Fisher

Introduction

The 'Culyer report' (Department of Health 1994) outlined the need for the delivery of care to be evidence-based and for health interventions to be subject to evaluation. Practitioners in new clinical roles are often engaged in both service development and delivery, and so are ideally placed to implement evidence-based care. Their proximity to patients/clients and their treatment offers them a very comprehensive picture of service use, which can then be used to provide reliable and accurate information to ensure that purchasing decisions are well informed. Their unique position allows them to see the 'whole picture' (Schaefer 1991).

This chapter will explore how practitioners in new clinical roles can contribute to the development of a practice environment that is conducive to delivering evidence-based health care. It will also seek to clarify how such practitioners access research evidence, appraise it, integrate the findings into their practice and share them with the consumers of their services. Examples will be drawn from the author's background in cardiac care as a Cardiac Liaison Nurse, but the principles are generic and can be applied to practitioners undertaking new clinical roles in other disciplines.

Why use evidence-based care?

A key aim of many of the new clinical roles in nursing and the health-care professions (HCPs) should be the development and implementation of 'evidence-based practice'. This requires practitioners to have an understanding of research methods and audit procedures in addition to their clinical expertise. In the past nurses and HCPs frequently failed to base their practice on research findings and often adopted a ritualistic approach to care. This is no longer defensible, especially in a climate of increasing litigation (Carter 1996). Evidence-based practice requires the removal of rituals and the replacement of outdated practices with those founded on scientific research evidence.

What is evidence-based care?

It is not always clear in the literature and policy documents exactly what is meant by the term 'evidence-based practice', which is often used interchangeably with the term 'research-based practice'. 'Research-based practice' suggests that practice be developed solely on the results of research findings in general, and of randomised clinical trials (RCTs) in particular, the so-called 'gold standard' of research methods. RCTs have traditionally been the dominant research method used in health care, and they have been used very effectively to investigate the effects of new drug therapies before their introduction into clinical practice. RCTs on their own, however, offer a limited means of building effective health services because they reflect only one facet of that service: namely, medical treatment. An effective health service is dependent on more than merely ensuring that the client receives the appropriate medical treatment. Therefore a broader approach to evidence-based practice is needed, which can incorporate findings from qualitative and quantitative research, audit results, activity data, and feedback from both service users and other members of the multidisciplinary team.

The provision of evidence-based care is the responsibility of both those who commission health care and those who deliver it (Deighan & Boyd 1996). Delivering evidence-based care requires the integration of clinical expertise with research findings (Sackett et al 1996). It is an approach to problem-solving in clinical practice, which involves the following:

◆ identifying the problem
◆ asking questions
◆ searching the literature (Rosenberg & Donald 1995)
◆ deciding which intervention to adopt, based on the available evidence (White 1997).

New clinical roles as a catalyst for the development of evidence-based health care

Practitioners in new clinical roles are well placed to act as a catalyst for the development of evidence-based health care (McSharry 1995). In fact, the climate of increasing specialisation in health care, coupled with an increased knowledge base, has been identified as the main reason for the development of nurse specialist roles (Castledine 1995). Practitioners in new clinical roles are close to service users and managers, and to other members of the multidisciplinary team with whom they can collaborate to ensure that appropriate and timely care delivery takes place. Their unique position enables them to influence the shape and content of services and the mode of delivery. Health professionals have grown accustomed to change being imposed from above (top-down), with little or minimal involvement (Smith & Masterson 1996). Practitioners in new clinical roles can provide a vital link between theory and practice (McSharry 1995) and prevent this happening.

Operationalising the new clinical roles

Clinical expertise within a specialty is vital for the development of evidence-based practice, as is an in-depth knowledge of research methods. Practitioners in new clinical roles must be able to review research findings critically and decide whether such findings are reliable and applicable to their area of practice. A working knowledge of audit methods is equally important as this allows practitioners to evaluate their work and the effects of any service innovation. It has been argued that practitioners in new clinical roles such as clinical nurse specialists should be educated to graduate level in order to fulfil the diverse requirements of such roles (American Nursing Association 1980, Humphris 1994). However, many practitioners undertaking new clinical roles in the UK do not possess degree-level qualifications. This may affect their ability to evaluate research literature critically and in an effective manner.

Practitioners in new clinical roles are not always actively involved in research, despite claims that this is an essential facet of the job (Schaefer 1991). This may be the result of a variety of factors including the need for practitioners to prioritise their work commitments more effectively, insufficient resources, a lack of education in research methodology and poor employer support. Role conflicts may arise if managers emphasise the importance of service delivery at the expense of 'softer' options such as education and research activities, which may be given a low priority by the organisation.

Whilst the ability to undertake original research may be limited, and may not even be desirable, practitioners in new clinical roles can act to develop and provide services that are evidence-based. It is important that their services incorporate reliable evidence and that this is made clear to their service managers. They should also disseminate and share this evidence with other colleagues. Their close proximity to practice affords a unique opportunity to apply research findings to their own area of work (Sutton & Smith 1995). Standards must be set against which their work can be audited and evaluated in the context of current research evidence (Humphris 1994). To do this, services need to have clearly defined boundaries and aims from which service standards can be produced. This will allow an audit framework to evolve in tandem with the service, so that all interventions can be assessed for their efficacy, as Box 3.1 demonstrates.

Recent government health initiatives outlined in 'Our healthier nation' (Department of Health 1998) and 'Saving Lives' (Department of Health 1999) have advocated an increasing role for primary care in service commissioning and provision. The macro-political philosophy has moved from one of competition to collaboration in patient/client care. It acknowledges widening inequalities in health, and encourages a focus on improving the health of those who are worse off with the aim of preventing avoidable illness. Implicit in these new government policies is a more holistic approach to tackling ill health requiring the identification of areas with poor health and social conditions and encouraging the formation of healthy alliances to tackle these inequalities. New clinical roles have much to contribute in this area. The main specialist

---

Box 3.1 Community-based Cardiac Liaison Nurse (CLN) service

Aims and objectives

◆ To work across the primary/secondary care interface to provide continuity of care for coronary heart disease (CHD) clients and their families, by developing a consistent approach towards client care

Areas of responsibility

◆ Clinical
Client group: those discharged from secondary/tertiary care following acute episode of CHD
Interventions: identification of symptoms; advice on treatments and lifestyle change
Detailed structure of clinical component: clients visited within 2 weeks of discharge

◆ Liaison
Between primary, secondary and tertiary care sectors, to promote communication between health professionals and seamless care

◆ Education
Provide education and training on aspects of CHD management for clients, local community groups and health professionals

◆ Research
Develop evidence-based service initiatives
Identify gaps in service provision and make recommendations for change
Evaluate service for purchasers

Information given regarding

◆ Diagnosis; treatments received/pending; medication; risk factor management; local rehabilitation services

Outcomes of visit

◆ Refer clients on to other specialist services as necessary, i.e. social services, clinical psychologist, cardiologists, rehabilitation nurses

◆ Clients will be given a written summary of the visit and a contact number for the Cardiac Liaison Nurse Service

◆ Written summaries will be sent to relevant health professionals within 24 hours of the visit

---

role within cardiac services has traditionally been that of the cardiac rehabilitation nurse, whose focus has been on assisting individuals to return to normal after an acute cardiac event, whilst other more chronic aspects of living with heart disease have often been overlooked. However, new cardiac roles are also emerging in occupational therapy and physiotherapy (School of Health and Related Research 1999).

Using the example of the Cardiac Liaison Nurse Service, the client group, the location of the service and four main areas of responsibility are identified within Box 3.1, which provides practitioners with a template on which to build their services. It outlines when the client will be visited, what will happen during the visit and what the possible outcomes of the visit will be. Once parameters such as these have been set then an audit framework can be developed to see whether these aims have been met or not. If any of these are not achieved, it is important to investigate why, because issues from outside the service may also have an impact on its effectiveness. Research is important in providing the evidence base for the services delivered and in evaluating them to see how effective or otherwise they are.

Issues in role evaluation

Cardiac rehabilitation programmes have often been focused on exercise and lifestyle and have usually been evaluated in terms of numbers of patients seen and the modification of risk factors such as blood pressure and weight. Whilst these traditional exercise-based programmes increase physical well-being, they do not actually increase survival (Hampton & McWilliam 1992). Many individuals will return to their former activities quickly even if they only follow the information given to them at time of discharge.

Cardiovascular disease (CVD) is the major cause of premature morbidity and mortality in the United Kingdom and is a major drain on NHS finances (Department of Health 1998). However, it is not seen as a chronic and malignant disease, unlike cancer, and consequently there are far fewer new roles within the specialty in comparison to cancer. Generally the emphasis in cardiac care is on active treatment and 'curative' interventions such as coronary artery bypass grafting, which masks the chronic nature of the condition. Consequently, cardiac rehabilitation services focus on rehabilitating individuals after acute episodes such as myocardial infarction and their effectiveness is measured in terms of the physical risk factors modified.

Evaluation tends to be very limited and in this context is more suited to acute illnesses rather than a malignant condition. This reflects a culture of 'short-termism', a culture that expects quick results and which often affects the funding of such posts. It is not uncommon to see new posts being developed with funding for 2–3 years, during which time the practitioner will have to demonstrate that the services offered are effective. It is not surprising therefore that alterations in physical measurements such as blood pressure reduction, weight reduction and effective blood sugar control are often chosen as these can be easily identified and measured and levels can change within a relatively short time span. Consequently, practitioners may find themselves developing initiatives that only confer a short-term benefit to the client. Restricting evaluation of these services by the use of short-term indices alone does not assess how or if such changes are maintained over time, or investigate the psychological impact of such programmes.

Another difficulty for practitioners wishing to demonstrate the efficacy of their service is trying to isolate their input into a client's care from that of other members of the multidisciplinary team. Box 3.2 sets out the wide range of people that may come into contact with a client, all of whom may provide information and advice. Very few practitioners work in total isolation from other health-care professionals. Effective cross-boundary working requires a high level of interaction and collaboration between health professionals across the primary/secondary care divide (Hibberd 1998). The cardiac liaison nurse, for example, is required to promote effective communication across the primary/secondary care interface and between different health professionals who may not normally communicate with each other. This highlights the importance of evaluating all of the aspects of new clinical roles rather than just client outcomes in order to reflect the totality of the impact of the role.

Evaluating services

Evaluation can be more straightforward if an audit trail is set up at the same time as the role itself is developed. This allows practitioners to assess their practice and activity on a continuous basis, from the beginning. Unfortunately, because the main focus of many new clinical roles is the delivery of the clinical service itself, there is a danger of focusing time and resources on developing this at the exclusion of all else. Admittedly service activity can only be audited if it has been operational for some time. However, attempts to audit services retrospectively often fail to deliver any meaningful results, as postholders may not have defined what it is that they wish to measure or evaluate and what data should be collected for such purposes. By deciding this early on in any new role the practitioner allows appropriate data to be collected in a useful format from the start and helps identify any potential problems with the data collection method or findings early, so that modifications may be made.

What information should practitioners collect?

Information should be collected from a variety of sources if practitioners are to show evidence of their effectiveness (Table 3.1).

Collecting information from clients and their carers about the impact of the service they have received is vital, but caution is needed when interpreting the results due to the 'halo' effect which can occur when clients discuss

Box 3.2 Number of people who offer information to individuals suffering a myocardial infarction

Scenario
An 58-year-old woman is admitted to an acute cardiac care area with a diagnosis of acute myocardial infarction. The nurse admitting her identifies the following risk factors:

◆ A diet high in saturated animal fats
◆ Smoking history of 15 cigarettes a day for 40 years
◆ Sedentary lifestyle
◆ 2 stone overweight

Nursing assessment

◆ Client has a knowledge deficit about the nature and causes of CHD and is very anxious about the severity of her condition and how it may affect her life in future

Areas requiring intervention

◆ Knowledge deficit re: CHD and possible risk factors
◆ Action and effects of medication
◆ Treatments
◆ Lifestyle advice and information
◆ Anxiety and fear of the future

Individuals who may have an input

◆ Accident and emergency staff
◆ Ward nurses
◆ Ward medical team
◆ Cardiac rehabilitation nurse
◆ Consultant
◆ Outpatient department staff
◆ Other patients
◆ General practitioner
◆ Practice nurse or receptionist
◆ Family members and friends
◆ Cardiac liaison nurse

health professionals (Notter 1995). This can be at least partially overcome by delaying the collection of information until some time has elapsed from the intervention. It can also be minimised by collecting the information

Table 3.1 Sources of information for service evaluation

Source	Information to collect	Questions	Information obtained
Service users			
Clients	Demographic data Age Sex Ethnic group Socio-economic group Area of residence	How were clients contacted? Was the visit beneficial? Was there anything that should have been included/omitted?	Demographic data allows for stratification of results and targeting of specific intitiatives to specific groups Client perspective and evaluation of service can highlight areas for change
Health professionals	Category, e.g. General practitioner District nurse Health visitor Hospital consultant Cardiac rehabilitation nurse Local community groups	What contact have they had with the CLN Service (e.g. educational) Client referral to/ from service Have summaries been sent? Was the content of use? Are there any areas for change?	Can identify main sources and reasons for referral Can evaluate effectiveness of service from different health professional perspectives
Other sources			
Practitioner notes	Documentation of all stages of clinical service from initial referral to discharge Client demographic data		Can obtain raw activity data from notes and compare with findings from service users

anonymously, e.g. via a postal questionnaire; this is often preferable to a face-to-face meeting at which clients may find it difficult to express their true thoughts and feelings. In the case of the Cardiac Liaison Nurse Service, the Clinical Audit Department acted as a neutral third party, sending out a client questionnaire 6 months after the practitioner interventions, and collating and analysing the results.

Any audit/evaluation information should be shared and fed back to the relevant stakeholders so that they are aware of how the role is evolving. This is vitally important where the role is a new one or where the role operates across boundaries or specialties. Peer review can also promote an effective, systematic, critical and continuous reflection on performance (Grol 1994). This also provides an opportunity for stakeholders to make comments about possible changes in service delivery. Teamwork is desirable for effective audit to occur and support from audit staff is particularly important for clinicians in the primary care setting to assist them in identifying the appropriate areas for audit and to select criteria and standards (Hearnshaw et al 1994).

Littlejohn et al (1996) highlighted the fact that nurses are often concerned about their ability to influence purchasers' contracting decisions, which means that key decisions regarding service delivery may be made without adequate specialist input. Practitioners in new clinical roles need to be proactive; otherwise they may be restricted to providing services decided by the purchasers with only minimal practitioner input. By increasing their access to those involved with service planning and provision and by providing research-based evidence demonstrating what their role entails and achieves, they can help inform the decision-making process (Notter 1995). Box 3.3 provides examples of cross-boundary working in a Cardiac Liaison Nurse Service.

The Cardiac Liaison Nurse (CLN) provided specialist nursing input for clients with CVD across a health authority. This involved liaising with staff from three acute hospitals and all the general practitioners and community health practitioners within the specified health authority. Each of these groups was

---

Box 3.3 Care areas covered by the Cardiac Liaison Nurse Service

Tertiary care (1 centre)
◆ Cardiothoracic services

Secondary care (2 centres)
◆ General medicine
◆ Cardiology
◆ Care of the elderly

Primary care
◆ General practitioners (75 practices)
◆ Practice nurses
◆ District nurses (4 localities)
◆ Health visitors (4 localities)

included in the service audit and the collated findings were disseminated to each group, to promote effective communication and enhance collaboration between them and the practitioner. Sharing information with colleagues and being accessible in these ways can also promote the use of the practitioner as an educational and practice resource.

How to collect information

Practitioners in new clinical roles require many skills to fulfil all the requirements demanded of them. The obvious focus of their role is the provision of expert care, but their ability to demonstrate the value of this care is also important. Not all practitioners will have expertise or experience in using information technology (IT) resources or developing audit trails. To do this requires effective collaboration, in particular with the audit department (if there is one) and IT support. These experts can help practitioners to identify suitable audit tools and assist them in the collection of activity data reliably and quickly.

Setting up an audit

Practitioners should be evaluating their role and the delivery of their service regularly and any changes they may make in light of changing research evidence should also be monitored. Some of the questions the practitioner needs to answer in such reviews include:

◆ Who is the service being delivered to?
◆ How is it being delivered?
◆ Is the service targeting the appropriate client group?
◆ Does the actual service delivery match the proposed service delivery?
◆ Is the content of the service appropriate and relevant? Is it evidence-based?
◆ Is it meeting the needs and expectations of other health professionals?
◆ What impact is it having on the client's health status?
◆ What are the effects of any changes that have been made, in response to earlier audit findings?

This list is by no means exhaustive, but it can give a focus to the audit process and provide a baseline from which to initiate an audit. Audit requires the collection of both quantitative data regarding patient contact and qualitative data to capture the patient/client experience. The use of routine activity data for audit and evaluation purposes is recommended because it is cheap, no extra costs are incurred in its collection and time trends can easily be identified as the data is updated.

Table 3.2 Common pitfalls when setting up a service audit

No definition of how the service is actually delivered	Have not identified steps undertaken from initial referral to discharge
Lack of clear endpoints	Not sure what is being measured Too much information collected
Mismatch between what is to be measured and information collected	Using inappropriate measurement method or assessment tool
Attempt to audit service retrospectively	Information required has not been collected
Resource constraints	Not enough time available Not enough money available Lack of experience of setting up audit

In many instances practitioners in new clinical roles will be responsible for developing and implementing audit and analysing the results. Resources may be limited and the practitioner may be constrained particularly in terms of time available and costs. Table 3.2 highlights the common pitfalls.

Collaboration with the local audit department can avoid such pitfalls. Practitioners are usually able to describe the 'process' of their work but are often unclear about what the 'outcomes' are or how this is related to the process they have undertaken. Collaboration with the audit department can help identify key steps in the process, which can then be measured.

Practitioners may also have to collect and analyse their own audit and activity data and so they will need to have a quick, easy-to-use method of collecting data and collating it. Formulation of a grid based on service interventions is a quick and accurate method of collecting activity information and can be ticked off at the end of each consultation (Notter 1995). Questionnaires can be used to obtain information from service users about specific aspects of the service; however, collating these by hand is time-consuming, prone to error and limited in the types of analysis that can be performed.

The use of information technology for audit and activity analysis purposes

The use of simple computer resources such as a clinical activity database can aid the collection of accurate and up-to-date records of workload, client profiles, etc. The system needs to be easily accessible and straightforward to use. Again, discussion with IT staff may save a lot of time and effort. Ready

Table 3.3 Examples of information obtained from activity database

Field	Information collected
Patient details	Name, address Age, sex, ethnicity, occupational status Housing tenure
Consultant	Name, specialty
GP details	Name, address, fundholding status
Hospital stay details	Hospital name, date of admission, discharge
Medical information	Diagnosis, treatment
Medication	Types and dosages
Risk factors for cardiac disease	Cholesterol, smoking history, weight, etc.
Referral information	Who referred client, date referral received Date client contacted to arrange visit Date of visit
Summary	When summary written, mailing list

access to a personal computer is required. An activity database can be set up on a commercial database package, such as Microsoft Access©. The database can be designed to reflect the format of the written service documentation, which should reduce operator error when entering data. Data can be entered at the end of each day and week to provide an accurate archive of activity, which can be accessed easily and quickly. The use of a computerised database will also allow for more detailed analysis than can be gained from written notes.

Table 3.3 sets out the information kept on a database by the CLN. The left-hand columns represent fields in the database and those on the right give an indication of the content of each. The format of the database is designed to be identical to the nursing documentation used, so that the information can be entered directly without any further modification or coding. From this it is possible to obtain detailed profiles of clients.

The collection of information in this format allows more detailed analysis to be undertaken. For example, information on numbers of patients seen can be stratified by:

◆ sex
◆ age
◆ ethnic group
◆ occupational class

- ◆ area of residence
- ◆ diagnostic category
- ◆ interventions received.

This offers a much more detailed picture than just counting the total number of client visits over a particular period. This information can also help build up a detailed profile of who accesses the service most in terms of who makes the referrals and where they are located. Information on costs involved with any particular interventions should also be included where possible, as services are more likely to be adopted if they can be shown to be both research-based and cost-effective (Hicks 1997). Practitioners will need to work closely with their local finance department to try and apply costings to their services. Such detailed information can be fed back to service purchasers and key stakeholders and can be used to inform the service planning process at health authority and primary care group level. Practitioners themselves can also access activity data from such a database, which they can then compare against their service standards. For example, they could look at how many referrals they saw within the time stated in the service guidelines. Thus databases of this sort can also provide a useful form of professional benchmarking.

Sources of evidence

In the earlier part of this chapter I identified strategies to help practitioners in new clinical roles to function effectively and evaluate their service. I will now look at how practitioners can translate information from research evidence into their practice.

Library resources

Evidence-based practice cannot be developed if the evidence cannot be accessed by practitioners. Libraries are an obvious source of information and are invaluable for undertaking detailed literature searches. However, most libraries are based in higher education institutions; if they are hospital based, they are sometimes administered by the local university or access is restricted for non-medical staff. Unless practitioners are studying at the university in question, they may not be able to use the facilities or may have to pay a fee to do so. This situation is often exacerbated for community-based practitioners, who may be based in clinics or health centres.

Computer-based sources of information

Another source of information that is growing in both popularity and quality

Box 3.4 Some useful websites

The Cochrane Collaboration
On-line database of systematic reviews, regularly updated
Http://www.neuronet.org/cochrane.htm

NHS Centre for Reviews and Dissemination
Publish 'Effective health care bulletins'
Http://www.york.ac.uk/inst/crd/welcome.htm

Promoting Clinical Effectiveness
Booklet produced by NHSE to promote greater clinical effectiveness
Http://wwwjr2.ox.ac.uk/Bandolier/band25/b25-4.html

UK Nursing Sites
Web site linking nursing organisations and various special interest groups
Http://www.shef.ac.uk/~nhcon/nuuk.htm

NHS Nursing Home Page
Http://www.doh.gov.uk/nursing.htm

United Kingdom Central Council for Nursing, Midwifery and Health Visiting
http://www.ukcc.org.uk

Royal College of Nursing
http://www.rcn.org.uk

RCN Library
http://www.rcn.org.uk/library/library.htm

World Health Organization Nursing
http://www.who.int/hdp/nur

is that provided by the Internet. Journals can be accessed electronically, as can a number of national databases dealing with the dissemination of clinical evidence (see Box 3.4). This medium can also be used as a method of bringing interested parties together to share and exchange information. Indeed it may become the ideal method of networking for practitioners who find it difficult to meet each other due to shift/work commitments. Not only does it allow colleagues to network locally and nationally but it can also be a means of establishing contacts with colleagues internationally. Practitioners can use the Internet to access information and discuss work-related issues without leaving the workplace and this can be a boon for health professionals who traditionally have difficulties in being released from clinical duties to pursue 'soft, low-priority' research activities.

Appraising research evidence

Whatever its source, practitioners need to decide whether the information obtained is reliable or valid. Appraising research evidence can be a lengthy and complex process. There are a number of health-related Internet sites, which may be of interest to practitioners who are committed to evidence-based practice (see Box 3.4). These provide summaries of systematic reviews of published research on a variety of topics, and comment on the reliability of the findings and methodologies used. Many of the reports can be accessed directly from the websites or can be purchased for a reasonable fee.

Sharing ideas and information

NHS Trusts should have clear strategies for disseminating information amongst health professionals, and these should be dynamic, to reflect the changing context of care delivery, rather than prescriptive (Haines & Jones 1994). In the example of the Cardiac Liaison Nurse Service, annual evaluation meetings were arranged with interested stakeholders, where audit and activity data were presented because this type of collaboration is likely to assist in the dissemination of information (Moores 1996).

Executive members of the local community Trusts, health authority purchasers and key stakeholders from acute Trusts were invited to these meetings so that findings could be presented and discussed in an open forum. This data was also presented to the local acute hospital Trust audit meetings, so that the collaborative nature of the service was emphasised and to allow Trusts to change practices in response to the findings if indicated.

Publication of findings is a useful channel for sharing information with other colleagues and has the potential to reach a wide audience (Smith & Masterson 1996). Access to on-line resources can also provide a valuable communication link with other health-care professionals and promote effective networking and sharing of information and ideas.

Practitioners may find it difficult to arrange time to attend conferences and study days or to share information with their peers, due to clinical commitments and pressures. Computer resources can be a very effective medium to support such activity. The rapid development of the Internet and e-mail allows practitioners to stay in touch with colleagues all over the world without leaving their clinical area. If the resources are available, practitioners could have a web page devoted to their service, outlining the service's aims and objectives and providing a contact address for interested parties. This is likely to become more commonplace as computer technology becomes more widely implemented within health-care settings.

Such resources can also allow the practitioner to develop effective communication with her employers and stakeholders, e.g. reports of service activity can be circulated by e-mail instantaneously, and can then be accessed almost immediately. This reduces costs and delays in copying and posting documents. Communication becomes fast and efficient and stakeholders are kept informed. Providing accurate up-to-date information in this way is likely to lead to more informed purchasing decisions. Paper-based systems suffer from a built-in time delay due to the time taken to gather and analyse information from them. This can lead to commissioning decisions being made on inaccurate and out-of-date information which may not reflect current practice.

Computer skills

Practitioners are expected to be clinical experts, and this is often the only prerequisite for employment. Definitions of what is required to be an effective practitioner in a new clinical role tend to focus on clinical expertise and academic attainment with little discussion about the skills practitioners actually require to do their job. The ability to carry out and use audit findings is a fundamental part of the evaluation of such roles. The possession of IT skills will become increasingly important as information and communication technology becomes faster and more reliable. Computer and IT skills can enable the following:

◆ secretarial and administrative support
◆ archiving for service and audit data
◆ access to on-line information: clinical journals, review databases
◆ communication tool: e-mail.

Lack of basic IT skills will seriously hinder the ability of practitioners to perform their role effectively. Paper-based systems may be reassuring due to their familiarity, but they are inefficient in terms of storage, accuracy and retrievability. Computer-based systems take up less storage space and are more accurate. Data can be retrieved from them quickly and in a variety of formats, which can help the practitioner be more flexible and save a great deal of time. Helping practitioners gain IT skills will often require the development of a close working relationship with the IT support staff. The support required may be intensive at the outset, but with time may develop into more of an advisory and troubleshooting role.

Problems in evaluation

Having identified a framework for successful role development I will now explore the problems which may be encountered when practitioners try to evaluate the services they offer, or specific aspects of them. By their very nature, most new clinical roles involve cross-agency working and collaboration and it can be impossible to identify which particular health professional was responsible for any given identifiable health outcome. Sackett et al (1996) see effective evidence-based care as being multidisciplinary and yet many practitioners are expected to evaluate their role without accounting for the input made by other health professionals. Arguably, practitioners working in new clinical roles should be aiming to promote their role as a catalyst for multidisciplinary working in order to provide their service users with 'seamless care'.

Unfortunately in the drive to demonstrate their effectiveness practitioners often attempt to isolate fragments of their work which either do not reflect the totality of their role or produce meaningless figures. This means that it can be very difficult for employers to identify whether their practitioners are effective or not, or whether they are using resources effectively. Yet the ability of practitioners in new clinical roles to demonstrate their economic viability is of paramount importance in a health service that is struggling to contain costs (Heasell 1996).

In Box 3.5, again using the Cardiac Liaison Nurse Service as an example, the

---

Box 3.5 Individuals who may have input into care/recovery

Inpatient phase
◆ Medical staff
◆ Nursing staff
◆ Rehabilitation nurse
◆ Cardiologist
◆ Friends and family
◆ Other patients

Post-discharge phase
◆ Friends and family
◆ Rehabilitation nurse
◆ General practitioner
◆ Practice nurse
◆ Cardiac liaison nurse
◆ Members of cardiac rehabilitation group
◆ Outpatient medical and nursing staff

individuals who may have input into a client's recovery and rehabilitation from an acute coronary event are identified. Part of the CLN's role is to work closely with other health professionals and family members, so it can be difficult to identify which of these individuals may be responsible for the client making a particular change in his lifestyle or behaviour.

A desire to see results quickly, which may be driven by the short-term funding of some projects as outlined earlier, may also cause problems. Practitioners are forced to develop services that will produce quick results, at the expense of developing services which may produce long-term health gains. For example, practitioners may be able to demonstrate that their interventions have led a client to modify her behaviour but may not be able to identify whether this change is maintained or not. In addition, such evaluation designs may neither acknowledge the collaborative aspects of care nor reflect the multifactorial nature of many conditions such as CHD. They also encourage a heavy emphasis on direct treatment-related outcomes which do not sit easily within a broader paradigm of health promotion and may reflect the dominance of the medical approach to care and service delivery. Such approaches do not reflect the chronic nature of many health problems where alleviation of symptoms and improved quality of life may be more appropriate outcomes than cure.

This reflects concerns voiced by clinicians that an over-reliance on evidence-based care is a method of introducing cost-cutting, with the emphasis solely on producing cost-effective care (Deighan & Boyd 1996). Whilst evidence-based care should allow for a more effective use of scarce resources, practitioners may uncover inappropriate or subtherapeutic interventions which may not be cost-effective to rectify. For example, the CLN service uncovered a significant number of clients with elevated blood lipids, who were not on appropriate medication in the form of statins for their cardiac conditions. In this case the most effective treatment is not cheap and such interventions need to be incorporated into policy decisions (Deighan & Boyd 1996).

Clinical guidelines

Practitioners in new clinical roles can also help develop an evidence-based practice culture through assisting in the development of best-practice guidelines, which could be used to direct other practitioners to deliver evidence-based care. Properly developed clinical guidelines can change practice and lead to changes in patient outcomes (Deighan & Boyd 1996). However, there are legal considerations because guidelines may not be legally defensible. Clinical discretion must be exercised, as a treatment not described in a guideline may be required by a client and should not be withheld solely on the grounds that it does not appear in the guideline. Standardisation of practice must be looked on with caution, as the health status of clients is dynamic and health-care delivery is not in itself an exact science (Tingle 1996). Successful guidelines are developed collaboratively by a multi-disciplinary team of stakeholders involved in care delivery (Duff et al 1996).

Conclusion

This chapter has examined how practitioners in new clinical roles can promote the development of a practice environment that is conducive to implementing evidence-based practice. This reflects current government policies that expect health-care interventions to be based on a sound research base and be subject to evaluation of their effectiveness. Practitioners have a responsibility to develop services based on sound evidence and the importance of audit to demonstrate this cannot be underestimated. The central role to be played by these practitioners has been identified. They are ideally placed, in close proximity to those who use their services and to those who commission services. Practitioners also have a duty to collect accurate service activity and audit data to demonstrate the efficacy of their own services and to provide this information to those responsible for commissioning new services. Expert practitioners can be close to those making decisions regarding clinical services and can actually influence service delivery and configuration. For practitioners in new clinical roles to fulfil the varied and disparate roles expected of them, i.e. experience of developing audit, multiprofessional working, translating research findings into meaningful practice, they may well require more skills than those offered in current education programmes.

REFERENCES

American Nursing Association (1980) Nursing: a social policy statement. ANA, Kansas City

Carter D (1996) Barriers to the implementation of research findings in practice. Nurse Researcher 4(2):30–40

Castledine G (1995) Defining specialist nursing. British Journal of Nursing 4(5):264–265

Deighan M, Boyd K (1996) Defining evidence-based health-care: learning strategy? NT Research 1(5):332–339

Department of Health (1994) Supporting research and development in the National Health Service. NHS R&D Taskforce (Culyer report). HMSO, London

Department of Health (1998) Our healthier nation. A contract for health. Stationery Office, London

Department of Health (1999) Saving lives: Our healthier nation. Stationery Office, London

Duff L, Kitson A, Seers K, Humphris D (1996) Clinical guidelines: an introduction to their development and implementation. Journal of Advanced Nursing 23:887–895

Grol R (1994) Quality improvement by peer review in primary care: a practical guide. Quality in Health Care 3:147–152

Haines A, Jones R (1994) Implementing findings of research. British Medical Journal 308:1488–1492

Hampton J, McWilliam A (1992) Purchasing care for patients with acute myocardial infarction. Quality in Health Care 1:68–73

Hearnshaw H, Baker R, Robertson N (1994) Multidisciplinary audit in primary healthcare teams: facilitation by audit support staff. Quality in Health Care 3:164–168

Heasell S (1996) Economics of evidence about nurse specialisation. British Journal of Nursing 5(16):991–994

Hibberd P (1998) The primary/secondary interface. Cross-boundary teamwork – missing link for seamless care. Journal of Clinical Nursing 7:274–282

Hicks C (1997) The dilemma of incorporating research into clinical practice. British Journal of Nursing 6(9):511–515

Humphris D (1994) The basis of role specialism in nursing. In Humphris D (ed) The clinical nurse specialist: issues in practice. Macmillan, Basingstoke

Littlejohn P, Dumelow C, Griffiths S (1996) Knowledge-based commissioning: can a national clinical effectiveness policy be compatible with seeking local professional advice? Journal of Health Services Research and Policy 1(1):28–34

McSharry M (1995) The evolving role of the clinical nurse specialist. British Journal of Nursing 4(11):641–646

Moores Y (1996) The research agenda: change, challenge, opportunity. NT Research 1(3):330–331

Notter J (1995) Marketing specialist practice to managers and purchasers. British Journal of Nursing 4(22):1330–1334

Rosenberg W, Donald A (1995) Evidence-based medicine: an approach to clinical problem-solving. British Medical Journal 310:1122–1126

Sackett D, Rosenberg W, Gray M et al (1996) Evidence-based medicine: what it is and what it isn't – it's about integrating individual clinical expertise and the best external evidence. British Medical Journal 312:71–72

Schaefer K (1991) Taking care of the caretakers: a practical explanation of clinical nurse specialist practice. Journal of Advanced Nursing 16:270–276

School of Health and Related Research (SCHARR) (1999) Exploring new roles in practice. SCHARR, University of Sheffield, Sheffield

Smith P, Masterson A (1996) Promoting the dissemination and implementation of research findings. Nurse Researcher 4(2):15–29

Sutton F, Smith C (1995) Advanced nursing practice: new ideas and new perspectives. Journal of Advanced Nursing 21:1037–1043

Tingle J (1996) Clinical guidelines: legal and clinical risk management issues. British Journal of Nursing 6(11):639–641

White S (1997) Evidence-based practice and nursing: the new panacea? British Journal of Nursing 6(3):175–178

4

Freedom to learn, freedom to be
Learning, reflecting and supporting in practice

Anne Palmer

'Experience is not what happens to you but what you make of what happens to you.'

Aldous Huxley

Introduction

It is a challenging time for those in new clinical roles as the complexities and chaos of individual practice are being continually tested by developing knowledge, new technologies, innovative treatments and the rising expectations of increasingly enlightened patient/client groups. It should be recognised, however, that the National Health Service (NHS) is not the only sector experiencing profound change as the effect of the information age impinges on the world of work and service delivery. The impact of global markets, increasing competition and the need for adaptability in the workplace has resulted in changing attitudes to work and work patterns. An increasing emphasis has been placed on the need for more flexible ways of working and learning (Department for Education and Employment 1995, 1996, Foster 1996). These changes include the development and application of:

◆ twilight shifts
◆ 24-hour working
◆ short-term contracts
◆ part-time working
◆ flattened management structures
◆ learning in the workplace.

These changes require individual workers to develop the appropriate abilities to adapt and become more 'customer' oriented. At the same time there is less job security due to the change in emphasis from full-time employment to part-time working and the advent of a new breed of worker, the 'just in-timers'. These individuals are employed for a short duration to fill a particular void in personnel or to provide specialist input for a specified contract (British Broadcasting Corporation 1999). In nursing and the health-care professions (HCPs), recruitment agencies are travelling ever further afield to attract international staff.

The result of these changes is a rapidly evolving workplace that is increasingly dependent on technology and the rapid dissemination of information. This brings with it the requirement for a workforce that is adaptable, knowledgeable, well skilled, up to date and able to respond to the changing needs and requirements of those they serve. It is a working context that those employed in new clinical roles such as clinical nurse specialists, physiotherapy practitioners and specialist radiographers will readily identify with.

The intention of this chapter is to reflect on the educational, support and developmental issues that impact on those who practise in new clinical roles. It is not my intention to join in the ongoing debates about the desirability or otherwise of such developments. Instead I wish to encourage careful consideration of the educational initiatives and learning support roles that currently exist. Consideration of this sort should enable practitioners and their managers to choose the programmes and practices that best fit their particular needs. It must be recognised that these needs will change depending on the personal and professional circumstances of the individual practitioners, the expertise they are developing and the context within which they practise. In identifying the range of strategies and roles available and the functions they perform, I hope that practitioners can be facilitated to select appropriate professional education, work-based learning approaches and clinical support to promote their learning in practice and enhance their personal and professional growth.

The current context of the new role developments in nursing and HCPs will be briefly discussed in making a case for these practitioners to become learning individuals. This will be followed by an exploration of the various perspectives on learning from experience, reflection in practice and the professional support roles that actively facilitate learning in practice. Finally the emerging issues for practitioners in new clinical roles will be discussed in relation to the contribution that learning organisations and learning societies can make in assisting the learning individual.

The current context

It would be easy to become embroiled in the healthy and interesting debate, which is currently engaging nursing and HCPs around the notions of advanced, specialist and 'higher-level practice'. It would also be easy to engage in retrospective reflection on how such a diversity of roles and responsibilities has emerged over the last decade or so. However, these topics are covered in other chapters. Useful additional sources which help to make sense of the historical developments and the current debates concerning diverse roles with similar titles but differing functions and philosophies include the beneficial text by Humphris (1994) and the newer and challenging tome produced by Rolfe & Fulbrook (1998).

Statutory body interest has also been recently stimulated with the United Kingdom Central Council for Nursing, Midwifery and Health Visiting (UKCC) engaging in an exercise to map out the issues and provide a coherent framework for the regulation of 'higher-level practice' in the professions it regulates. This is an exercise that should offer clarity and promote further dialogue concerning the current and future situation (UKCC 1998). The Chartered Society for Physiotherapy and the College of Occupational Therapists are also currently involved in similar work. In addition, the Secretary of state for Health has joined the debate in reporting that there should be fewer nursing grades, with those of Registered Practitioner, Senior Registered Practitioner and Consultant Practitioner (Department of Health 1999) having been identified for survival. The rationale being a need to reward such staff 'for the work they do and responsibility they carry' (Dobson 1999). Similar work is ongoing between the Department of Health and the HCPs' professional bodies regarding the grading of expert and leadership roles in these professions.

These new clinical roles should be grounded in clinical practice and postholders should be knowledgeable in their own field. Postholders should be able to draw together the range of educating, consultative, researching and policy-initiating subroles associated with such posts to benefit individual clients and further the development of clinical practice. They should also be able to act as a supportive guide, significant role model and consultant to others. In addition they should be able to move expertly between the various roles and responsibilities of practice as determined by individual, clinical, professional and cultural circumstances (Humphris 1994, Rolfe & Fulbrook 1998).

The drawing up of an effective framework for the development and regulation of new clinical roles will require recognition of the diversities and complexities of such roles that arise from specific local needs and individual Trust policies. Particular attention should be focused upon:

◆ the needs of the specialism
◆ the geographical area
◆ the individual practitioner's strengths and expertise.

It is imperative that such practitioners be developed and supported by existing and emerging learning approaches within appropriate professional support frameworks that assist individuals in:

◆ the development and integration of consultancy, education, policy implementation and research skills
◆ the articulation and critical appraisal of personal learning and self-direction
◆ the acknowledgement and appreciation of critical thinking and continual learning.

A variety of different types of learning strategy, education programme and supportive relationship are required which ensure appropriate personal and professional development in practice, allowing such practitioners to think for themselves, become self-directed and challenge the assumptions of the current working context.

The term 'learning approaches' as used here is taken to mean the experiential and reflective processes that are underpinned by critical thinking and the principles of adult learning (Boud et al 1985, Brookfield 1987, Cox 1992). Learning in this context concerns not just the absorption of knowledge, the changing of attitudes or the development of useful skills, it is also about being

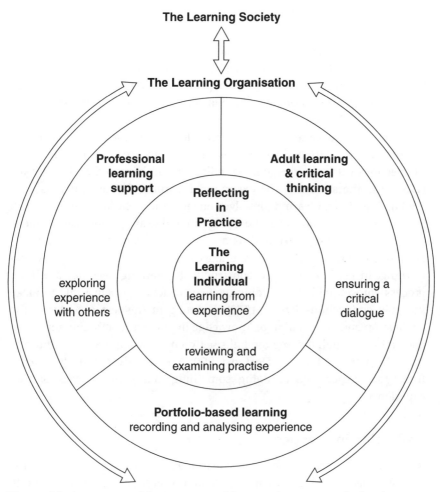

Figure 4.1 An overview of the integration of theoretical strategies and cultural perspectives involved in reflecting in practice

curious and developing self-confidence and self-awareness (Frazer 1992, Eraut 1994). It is therefore essential that a range of learning initiatives or approaches and professional support roles are considered that embrace these characteristics and meet the needs of those engaged in the 'swampy lowlands' of professional practice (Schon 1983) (see Fig. 4.1).

Freedom to learn: learning from experience by reflecting in practice

There is a growing recognition that learning involves building on our personal experiences as well as the people we work with, the resources we use, and the media activities we engage in, including surfing the Net (Miller & Boud 1996). Increasingly the focus for learning has moved from formal, classroom-based education programmes to recognising the importance of informal and incidental learning in the workplace (Marsick & Watkins 1990). This has resulted in a growing awareness of the importance of learning from experience in the practice domain.

Learning from experience or experiential learning is not a new concept but one that with the current drive towards reflective practice needs to be revisited. Connections with the emergence of reflection can be traced back to Dewey (1933) and the studies of the experiential learning theorists such as Kolb (1984). Experiential learning involves engaging in cycles of enquiry which lead to experimentation with the trying out and testing of ideas and actions in practice. Learning is viewed as a continuous process of re-evaluation, grounded in our own personal experiences which help us to appreciate that learning. In using experience constructively, learning becomes a vibrant process with individuals building new constructs and being able to make valuable connections (Freire 1978). Learning in this sense concerns the application and assimilation of knowledge in practice, combining reflection and action through making the links between 'knowing that' and 'knowing how' (Benner 84: 176). As Horton (1990: 57) so aptly puts it, 'you learn from your experience of doing something and your analysis of that experience.'

Reflecting in practice

Reflection, it is argued, facilitates learning from experience and assists professionals to work out what they do and what they need to learn and to make critical judgements on their effectiveness and efficiency (Schön 1983, Boud et al 1985, Cox 1992). Reflection and reflective practice in nursing and other HCPs have been in vogue for some time now as the original works of Schön (1983), Benner (1984) and latterly Johns & Freshwater (1998) have stimulated the consciousness of educators and practitioners seeking new ways to understand and appreciate the somewhat elusive practice of health care.

In reflecting in practice practitioners seek to derive meaning from new experiences which leads on to new perspectives and new ways of working (Atkins & Murphy 1993). Reflection allows individuals to 'capture their experience, think about it, mull it over and evaluate' (Boud et al 1985: 19). This, they suggest, will lead to new understandings, insights and actions, supporting Johns' (1998: 2) view that 'through reflective practice the practitioner may come to see the world differently, and based on these new insights may come to act differently.' Reflective practice, it is also suggested, assists in maintaining or improving the quality of care by encouraging self-awareness and critical appraisal (Palmer et al 1994).

Reflection then is the part of the learning process that allows us to find meaning within practice, to make sense of the world around us and to build on what is happening. However, it is more than practitioners working from personal experience, recalling what has happened, sharing their feelings with others, recording their observations as they review the experience, and exploring new meanings. Schön (1983), from his study of a variety of disciplines, has identified two processes: reflection-on-action and reflection-in-action. These two important processes may be at the heart of becoming what Rolfe (1998) terms a 'reflexive' practitioner. Rolfe also draws our attention to a deficiency in the nursing literature on reflective practice, claiming that it focuses predominantly on reflection-on-action techniques to the detriment of reflection-in-action. Reflection-on-action is reflection on an experience after the event. For example, Fitzgerald (1994) has clearly defined it as 'the retrospective contemplation of practice undertaken in order to uncover the knowledge used in a particular situation, by analysing and interpreting the information recorded'. Reflection-in-action, on the other hand, is reflecting on an experience while it is happening. This is a reflexive process – that is, one that changes the nature of the event as it is occurring.

To gain new insights and to contemplate new ways of acting, reflection, by its very nature, has to be more than a review or recall of experience. It also involves, as Van Menen (1990) has identified, a series of analytical processes whereby people develop capabilities to think actively (mindful); gain an awareness of what is happening (active); consider a range of possible actions and interventions (anticipatory); and contemplate the outcomes of such actions and interventions (recollective). These processes are well demonstrated by Johns' (1998) constructive model of structured reflection. This model facilitates the recording and analysis of experience through guided reflective cues. The beauty of this model is that it extends beyond the factual, personal, ethical and affective domains and enters the realms of reflexivity by encouraging connection with other experiences, resulting in a deeper analysis of any consequences.

Models such as Johns' may go some way towards offering a framework to assist practitioners in critical reflection and help them to move beyond the rhetoric of 'but we already do that' – when what they are commonly engaged in is a factual review of events (Wilson & Palmer 1998). The repeated phrase 'but we already do that' has to be recognised as rhetoric emerging from a practice culture that continues to focus on the 'doing', a culture whereby reflection is not readily valued and is seen as remaining within the domains of the academics and educators. It should be acknowledged that reflection, by its very nature focusing on the self, is not an easy process, particularly if practitioners are ill prepared and do not understand the implications for themselves and their practice. It requires a certain amount of fortitude to deal with what may be explored, the issues that may emerge and the 'messiness' of practice that may appear.

Other limiting aspects are included in what Boud & Miller (1996) classify as barriers to reflection. A full consideration of these is beyond the scope of this chapter, but their deliberations are well worth exploring because they identify barriers that appear to fit well with the current health-care climate and barriers that surface in the professional literature at regular intervals. These barriers include lack of time, external pressures and demands, and established patterns of thought and behaviour (Boud & Miller 1996: 79).

Exploring and analysing personal experiences requires a focus on self and the critical examination of practice. This may result in anxieties and insecurities about both, and allow the exposure of normal coping mechanisms (Graham et al 1998). This is where finding appropriate critical friends through effective professional support relationships is important and these will be discussed later in the chapter.

The reflective practitioner

How then can reflection – as the theorists have perceived it – be translated for the more pragmatic of us? How do we go about this reflecting and mulling over, within Schön's (1983) sense that 'the knowing is in our doing'? What we require is an appreciation of adult learning and critical thinking skills, which are vital in forming the basis for developing the relevant expertise to help practitioners think and act reflectively. An appreciation of these aspects of learning will facilitate the mature responses and analytical processes that underpin the practicalities of both reflection-in-action and reflection-on-action.

The practicalities of reflection-in-action and reflection-on-action involve:

◆ reviewing and examining your own practice
◆ having a critical dialogue with yourself
◆ maintaining and analysing a record of experiences and significant learning
◆ exploring personal experiences with others.

Such practicalities ensure that the emerging reflective practitioner not only gains new insights but generates new knowledge through experimentation and critical dialogue (Weil 1997, 1998, Rolfe 1998). These reflective and reflexive capabilities are often seemingly inherent within the roles and responsibilities of those aspiring to practise at a 'higher level'.

Reviewing and examining your own practice

Reviewing and examining your own practice is an essential aspect of working as an autonomous practitioner with responsibilities for your own client group. It involves a critical analysis of your everyday work, role and responsibilities from a personal perspective. It is also a sound idea and good practice if you invite others to become involved, as the value of peer assessment is highly recommended (Boud 1995, Gibbs 1995). Feedback and constructive comment from peers can provide new insights as well as recognition for the value of your role in the health-care team.

Reviewing and examining practice is necessary:

◆ as part of our professional responsibilities
◆ to justify role, functions and capabilities
◆ to provide opportunities for role development and attract resources
◆ to promote opportunities for creativity and innovation in practice
◆ to encourage individual development, self-awareness, a spirit of enquiry and personal value.

Reviewing involves identifying significant learning experiences or learning opportunities that have meaning for you personally. Examining these events is concerned with exploring the importance or value of what has occurred, or is occurring, in a systematic manner. Limitations and challenges can be examined and it is important to consider the feelings and attitudes that are apparent or emerge. Critical incident analysis based on Flanagan's (1954) original work is often cited as an effective framework for such explorations. Crouch (1991) suggests a series of open-ended questions to encourage analysis and Johns' (1998) structured model of reflection, as mentioned earlier, offers a constructive set of reflective cues.

In essence reviewing and examining practice should include an analysis of:

◆ What is happening?
◆ Who is involved?
◆ What am I feeling?
◆ What have I learnt?
◆ What will I do differently?

It is also useful to undertake activities that assist in the discovery of your own abilities and personal talents. This can be achieved by exploring important aspects of significant life events and career developments. It is also beneficial to maintain an inventory of the skills and attributes that make you unique. Such analysis will ensure learning becomes part of the survival strategy that equips practitioners with the intellectual abilities, clinical competence and strategic overview to provide client-centred quality care (Cameron 1994). It is also important when examining your own practice to embrace the other critical approaches that have gained credence in recent years, of which critical appraisal, critical reading and critical thinking have become the best known. The differences are documented in Clarke & Croft (1998) and other erudite texts that extol the virtues of study skills for health professionals. However, critical thinking is chosen for consideration here as it forms a vital part of adult learning, in ensuring critical reflection and in questioning yourself and your practice.

Having a critical dialogue with yourself

Engaging in a personal critical dialogue prepares practitioners for the discourse that occurs with others such as peers, other health-care practitioners, mentors and supervisors. It allows you the personal space to question what you are doing and how you are doing it, within a sense of knowing what you are doing. This brings meaning and context to each learning experience and in challenging yourself you are prepared for the times when others may challenge you.

Adult learning arises from the explorations of experiential learning and in particular the theoretical perspectives of Rogers' (1969) developmental strategies that there should be a 'freedom to learn'. This is complemented by the work of Knowles (1975, 1978) in providing the principles of how adults learn. A central feature of adult learning is that each individual becomes self-directing and plays an active part in the learning process. Adult learners seek their own directions, discover their own learning resources and take responsibility for the consequences of their actions (Rogers 1969). Adult learning shifts the emphasis away from didactic teacher-centred, content-driven initiatives towards activities that have meaning for the learner and require problem-solving skills. This facilitates learner autonomy and the further development of critical thinking skills. As previously discussed, it has long been acknowledged that experience, self-discovery and personal growth are important aspects of adult learning. Adult learners use a range of abilities and activities to take an active part in learning and in making sense of that learning; the learning process itself becomes a valued event that assists individuals 'to comprehend, understand and experience the world about them' (Ramsden 1992: 47).

Becoming an adult learner means:

◆ identifying yourself in the learning process
◆ becoming self-directed and self-motivated
◆ being responsible for your own learning and actions
◆ seeking appropriate resources to continue learning
◆ being able to solve problems.

Self-directed learning will only be successful if practitioners are facilitated to identify their own learning needs and set realistic aims and outcomes. There also has to be a continual commitment to learn within the notion that we are human beings not human 'doings', supporting the freedom to learn perspective in providing the freedom to discover yourself. Taking responsibility for learning rests also on the set of underlying principles that we began to tease out earlier in the discussions on experiential learning. These principles enforce the fact that learning involves both formal and informal opportunities, that there are different ways of knowing and that understanding your motivation to learn is integral to becoming self-directed. As part of the process of taking responsibility for learning there is also a need for practitioners to have an appreciation of what is meant by quality learning. This recognition of the need to identify quality learning reflects the change in emphasis from that of previous theoretical perspectives which focused on the quality of the teaching. Instead the onus is placed firmly on the learner. Having such an appreciation, the learner can make an informed decision about each learning opportunity (both formal and informal) that is offered or presents itself.

Quality learning involves:

◆ respect for scholarship
◆ knowing how to learn
◆ becoming a lifelong learner
◆ the ability to formulate an argument
◆ a desire to know more
◆ the ability to integrate knowledge
◆ the skills of critical analysis.

In taking an adult learning approach, practitioners can begin to set their own agendas and directions for learning and begin to formulate personal strategies that will make the most of each experience. At the heart of the adult learning enterprise is the ability to think critically, which requires practitioners to be open to alternative ways of examining their work and confident in their abilities to analyse their actions. As part of this process it is important to engage in a critical dialogue with yourself by challenging your assumptions and acknowledging that you are an adult learner. It involves discovering a sense of yourself within the health-care team as someone who is respected and valued, and has a contribution to make.

Critical thinking is the consideration of 'the assumptions underlying our and others' ideas and actions, and contemplating alternative ways of thinking and acting' (Brookfield 1987, p. x). The crucial elements of learning to think critically lie in the exploration and continual challenging of assumptions that lead to the active responses of contemplating alternative ways of thinking and acting. To foster a critical thinking approach, practitioners are required to become more questioning and more active in controlling their working environment. Brookfield (1987) recommends that, in wanting to think critically, it is the individual's responsibility to:

◆ identify and challenge assumptions because it is healthy to examine assumptions and the validity of ideas, values and beliefs
◆ imagine and explore alternatives because there are other ways of creatively looking at the world
◆ challenge the importance of context because the exploration of settings and situations results in new insights
◆ develop a healthy reflective scepticism because seeing is not always believing.

Essential to this process of critical and creative thinking is the development of an organisational culture where practitioners can:

◆ ask awkward questions
◆ engage in dialogue and discussion
◆ develop their creative ideas
◆ expect to question assumptions continually
◆ challenge and reshape the workplace
◆ review and reflect on their performance
◆ recognise and acknowledge responses and feelings
◆ take responsibility for their own actions.

Such a culture is found within organisations that are themselves continually learning and this will be discussed later within the remit of learning organisations. Becoming a critical thinker and an adult learner should not be a sterile academic endeavour that takes place in the classroom. It is much more concerned with the everyday management of practical experiences and the critical reflection on the experience that occurs. This ensures the development of creative ideas and facilitates a freshness and adaptability of approach to everyday work situations.

Maintaining and analysing a record of experiences and significant learning

Maintaining and analysing a record of experiences and significant learning is concerned with the writing up of the effects, implications and consequences of your experiences and reflections. It involves the documentation of personal feelings, behaviours and understandings of what has occurred and what is occurring. It is essential to record such deliberations as this allows situations and events to be reconsidered as new experiences and learning occur (Palmer 1996).

In nursing and the HCPs the maintenance of portfolios and profiles has been advocated as the vehicle for such written thoughts and deliberations. Other professions are also steadily recognising the importance of structured records of achievements and learning that go beyond the conventional curriculum vitae (Pietroni & Palmer 1995, Greater London Post-Qualifying Education and Training Consortium 1997). The terms 'portfolio' and 'profile' tend to be used interchangeably but generally a portfolio is an all-encompassing document that covers a range of situations, critical incidents, personal reflections and career issues, while a profile provides a prepared snapshot of certain aspects of the portfolio that can be shared with others. The profile separates particular information for a particular purpose and specified audience (Brown 1995). However, as Hull & Redfern (1996) have noted, there is still confusion surrounding the way in which individuals, organisations and statutory bodies use the terms.

Keeping a portfolio as described here is an effective way of reviewing and analysing your personal deliberations and is fundamental to the development of portfolio-based learning. Portfolio-based learning also has its origins in the experiential learning and adult learning theories. It is considered a useful and appropriate way to stimulate reflection, being more than the regular recording of personal and professional events (Simosko 1991). It involves the active processes of analysis and working with the entries to discover new ways of looking at situations and challenging personal assumptions. As Jasper (1998) has said, it is a dynamic entity that, developed properly, can support learning in practice.

The practicalities of keeping a portfolio involve working with your entries using perhaps a critical incident analysis approach or some other form of structured questioning that takes you beyond just a description of a situation. It is important to examine and evaluate the experiences and identify significant learning needs that result from such activities. An action plan can then be developed for setting about achieving further experiences and putting the new learning into practice. This process is well documented in Jasper (1998) with a clear example drawn from her own experience. By recording, reflecting and making plans for further action within the portfolio it is possible to demonstrate your achievements clearly along with the learning that has stemmed from your experience.

Hints on keeping a portfolio

The portfolio is a personal document so choose a method of keeping your records, notes, ideas and reflections that suits your individual learning style and talents. You could try out different ways of recording your thoughts – for example, through the use of video or by electronic means on a personal computer. What is important is to be yourself and write what is significant to you, recording what you think and feel.

It is also essential that you:

1. create time to write regularly
2. are frank and honest in your entries
3. let your ideas flow
4. are creative in using diagrams, drawings, cuttings or symbols
5. work with your ideas by examining issues that surface
6. are spontaneous and use your own words for feelings and behaviours
7. identify significant learning and highlight this in some way
8. regularly review your portfolio, updating and discarding as necessary.

These practical hints can make portfolio writing interesting and instead of becoming a chore your portfolio will become an important part of your journey towards reflective practice. It is essential to remember that it is not just writing in your portfolio that is important, it is the continual critical analysis and reflection on what has been recorded that assist you in benefiting from your experiences.

Exploring personal experiences with others

In ensuring adult learning and critical thinking it is imperative that we seek out others to act as confidants and 'sounding boards' to enable us to be supported through a constructive dialogue. As providing professional support is integral to the whole idea of developing a learning individual, the types of support role and relationship will be considered later in the chapter.

Being able to explore experiences with others is recognised as an important aspect of reflection (Marrow et al 1997, Johns 1998, Morton-Cooper & Palmer 2000). It forms an integral part of reflection and assists learning from experience in allowing practitioners to voice and share their values, perspectives, responsibilities and challenges. It is suggested here that the role of the mentor in particular is suitable for those wishing to practise at a 'higher level'. However, recognition should be given to the various professional support roles currently available to all staff as these have relevance and will play some part in professional development at different stages of a practitioner's career.

Practitioners seeking support and guidance from others have to be sure about their own abilities and what they want from the relationship in terms of the particular functions they offer. As part of the reviewing and examining process described earlier and to assist learning from experience, it would seem sensible to explore what types of learning support are required. Finding suitable support is important, particularly in today's turbulent working environment (Hughes & Pengelly 1997). Practitioners in new clinical roles should seek professional support roles that are enabling relationships where respect, genuineness and trust between the respective partners can be developed.

Freedom to be: professional support roles and relationships in practice

A key question then emerges concerning the range of professional support relationships that is applicable and available to those engaged in new clinical roles. It is beyond the scope of this chapter to explore the range of professional support roles and relationships in detail so the focus will be on those roles and relationships that have stimulated much of the debate in recent years and apply to the discussions here. The roles and relationships selected to assist learning from experience and stimulate critical thinking within an adult approach are those of mentoring, preceptorship and clinical supervision. For practical definitions of these and an overview of other recognisable learning support roles and relationships, see Table 4.1. These terms and definitions will change as the debate concerning professional support roles and relationships continues and new interpretations emerge.

Table 4.1 An overview of professional support roles in practice

Term	Definition
Assessor	A professionally competent practitioner skilled to assess others
Clinical supervisor	An experienced practitioner providing a professionally supportive relationship that encourages a practitioner (the supervisee) to critically reflect on his clinical practice
Coach	A skilled practitioner providing learning opportunities and supportive intervention
Co-tutoring	Individual practitioners working together to assist each other's learning and provide mutual support
Mentor	An individual providing an enabling relationship that facilitates personal growth and professional career development
Peer, buddy	A colleague of equal status, forming a collaborative relationship that is mutually supportive
Preceptor	An identified experienced practitioner working with a colleague to provide transitional role support
Role model	An individual whose demonstrable behaviour assists learning by example

Reference: Morton-Cooper & Palmer (2000)

The professional support roles available

In today's busy health-care climate even the most independent of professional practitioners require support, someone to share ideas with, seek advice from, critically reflect with and to provide a safe environment where feelings can be explored (Morton-Cooper & Palmer 1993, Parsloe 1995, Redfern & Roy 1998). Professional support systems such as mentoring, preceptorship and clinical supervision all have a part to play as recent policy changes, practice developments and staff shortages impact on the world of health-care work.

The development of professional support systems or schemes that provide guidance and promote learning through and from experience is not new. In UK nursing, mentoring was given credence within the development of 'Project 2000' and preceptorship appeared as a distorted version of American support initiatives for those that had qualified. Clinical supervision has now become a hot issue for some health professionals. There are those who argue that, had mentoring been effectively explored prior to initiation in practice, the continued confusion of appropriate support roles would not have arisen (Morle 1990, Barlow 1991, Morton-Cooper & Palmer 1993).

The recent debates in each of the health-care disciplines have tended to focus more on the clarification of roles and functions and less on the specific needs of individual practitioners as they struggle to make sense of the relevant theoretical approaches. The medical profession, however, is beginning to learn from nursing's early mistakes and relative confusion, with the identification of clear principles and useful guidance for the role of mentors within continuing medical education (Standing Committee on Postgraduate Medical and Dental Education 1998).

Mentoring

There is increasing recognition of the need for mentoring relationships that provide practitioners with a critical friend who supports and guides them through the organisational, social and political networks of the world of work to provide effective learning support and professional development. Mentoring of this type provides an emotionally intense adult relationship that is dynamic and durable and which encourages creativity and risk-taking. Mentoring can also assist with professional development by facilitating critical reflection on practice (Durgahee 1988).

Mentoring provides a relationship that assists with career socialisation in its broadest sense. It is a relationship that emerges classically from enabling cultures and would appear to be eminently suited to the needs of those wishing to practise independently and at a 'higher level'. Classical mentoring can be separated out from more formal or contract mentoring in that it is naturally occurring. The individuals find themselves and the relationship is focused on individual needs and maintained by the self-selection of the mentor and mentee. Formal or contract mentoring is artificially contrived to benefit organisational needs and the respective partners are paired in a formal manner. Mentoring of a short duration and with inappropriate partners has been referred to as pseudo-mentoring (Morton-Cooper & Palmer 2000). Mentoring should be an actively enabling relationship where experiences are shared and critically explored though a partnership of mutual trust and reciprocity.

In facilitating learning from experience: mentors

◆ are supportive and encouraging
◆ help in identifying resources
◆ are stimulating and challenging
◆ assist in identifying and building on personal strengths
◆ encourage creativity in practice and learning
◆ offer constructive feedback.

Individuals practising in new clinical roles require professional support that enables them to make sense of the complexities of their clinical practice, assists their professional development and encourages lifelong learning. It would seem that mentoring in its classical sense appropriately meets these demands. The issue for such practitioners is how to locate significant others with the enabling characteristics required. These characteristics include the qualities of a critical friend as well as the ability to give time and make themselves accessible, and having confidence in their abilities to share their experiences and assist in the development of another. It may be that those working in new clinical roles can provide support frameworks between themselves. Certainly nurse practitioners, clinical nurse specialists and advanced/specialist practitioners from the HCPs are in a unique position to seek partnerships with their colleagues from other professions and benefit from the richness of interprofessional mentoring.

Preceptorship

As the introduction of mentoring in UK nursing was originally targeted at student nurses and has resulted in the emergence of pseudo-mentoring approaches, preceptorship has been adapted to fit the needs of qualified nurses. Preceptorship is aimed at those returning to practice, changing roles or taking on new roles. Despite evidence from the North American literature suggesting preceptorship for those learning to nurse, in the UK it has become synonymous with the notion of transitional role support and is seen as a clinically oriented relationship. The preceptor acts as a clinical resource providing support and assisting in the development of clinical skills. In such a manner an effective clinical environment is created to stimulate learning and increased appreciation of the challenges of changing roles and taking on extra responsibilities (Morton-Cooper 1998). It is a role that could be used to support practitioners from any discipline who are practising at a 'higher level' or in a non-traditional way in the initial stages of their career development and in learning their role. By being essentially clinically focused, however, preceptorship lacks the interpersonal, inter-relational and wider career development aspects of mentoring.

Clinical supervision

Clinical supervision has steadily evolved from the developments in and the therapeutic frameworks of mental health social work and the therapy professions. It was introduced to the nursing audience thorough the Allit case (Davies 1993, Clothier et al 1994), the 'Vision for the future' report (Department of Health 1993) and the deliberations of researchers and statutory bodies (Butterworth and Faugier 1992, UKCC 1996).

Various models and approaches have been developed in the different health professions, with those in nursing relying heavily upon the seminal work of Procter (1986), who has identified the supervisory role as developing, evaluating and providing supportive help in the form of emotional refreshment. This has been adapted in nursing terms to provide for a clinical relationship that facilitates the development of skills, provides supportive help and promotes exploration of organisational issues (Nicklin 1995). In the HCPs generally, clinical supervision has been more closely associated with the development of competence prior to registration. However, the emerging clinical supervisor role for all of the health professions is that of providing a supportive environment that allows the practitioner to reflect on and mull over clinical issues. Reflection is considered an integral part of clinical supervision (Fowler & Chevannes 1998), with Johns (1993) even going so far as to identify what he calls professional supervision which encourages reflective practice. This fits with Bond & Holland's view that clinical supervision is 'regular protected time for facilitated, in-depth reflection on clinical practice' (Bond & Holland 1998: 12). The overall aim of clinical supervision therefore is the provision of effective focused support that sustains and creatively develops quality practitioners in the field.

The potential differences

Mentoring relationships promote personal and professional development as well as encouraging creativity and risk-taking. Mentors also provide for longer-term organisational support and are suitable for supporting development in the wider sense of the professional culture, leadership skills and socialisation to a career. Preceptorship is more clinically oriented and focused towards short-term relationships with specified aims and outcomes in changing or extending roles. Although Hawkins & Shohet (1989) consider supervision to concern reflection in the personal, professional and practice domains, general nursing appears to have chosen a more clinically focused relationship. This type of relationship goes beyond the remit of a specific resource relationship (preceptorship) but is not as organisationally or professionally wide-ranging as mentoring. It is important to note that Bond & Holland (1998) urge us to consider mentoring, preceptorship and clinical supervision as extensions of each other rather than as unnecessary substitutes for each other. These relationships in their opinion will provide for 'a range of opportunities for guidance, learning and support which should reflect the different degree and complexity of the needs of the practitioner at different stages in their career development' (Bond & Holland 1998: 23). As clinical supervision currently emerges as a clinically focused and supportive relationship which encourages in-depth exchanges between practitioners to sustain and develop the individual (Butterworth & Faugier 1992), it begins to fit somewhere in the middle of the continuum between mentoring and preceptorship. This continuum was originally explored by Puetz (1985) and further developed by Morton-Cooper & Palmer (2000).

The practical choices in seeking effective professional support

Having identified and discussed the roles and relationships available to those wishing to seek support as they work in new clinical roles it is essential to consider the practicalities of deciding what relationship best fits particular needs. The practitioners involved need to consider the relationship they require and who best can fulfil that role. In making such a choice it is important for practitioners to reflect on who they can work well with and who they feel safe with. To develop a sound enabling relationship, as described earlier, it is imperative to select someone who will provide a supportive relationship and who is:

◆ freely accessible
◆ responsive to others
◆ trustworthy
◆ confident and competent in her own abilities
◆ able to command respect
◆ capable of encouraging critical reflection.

Making an informed choice can be relatively simple and straightforward, with practitioners starting with such questions as 'What support do I need?' and 'Who can provide this?'. However, it is advocated that a personal review and assessment of individual needs should be carried out in a more considered manner. To do this, the key reflective questions that practitioners should be asking themselves are:

◆ What strengths do I have and want to build upon?
◆ What limitations do I want to explore and work on?
◆ What assistance and support do I require?
◆ How can I get the support that I need?
◆ Who will best provide that support (in the short term/long term)?

These open and reflective questions will lead to practitioners identifying their own particular requirements and to link their needs more readily with their individual circumstances, which may be very varied. Careful consideration of questions such as these may well lead to the practitioner setting up a variety of relationships as their personal and professional circumstances change over time. For example, what may start as a preceptor relationship may gather depth and longevity with a shift towards a more career-oriented, enabling relationship which manifests as that of mentoring.

How can I support others?

This is the ultimate question to be asked eventually by all practitioners working in new clinical roles. It is particularly relevant in relation to mentoring where there is evidence to suggest that those who have been mentored are more likely to mentor others (Roche 1979, Palmer 1987). The same may eventually be true of the other professional support relationships but the evidence is not yet available. The hope is that, by creating and encouraging sound supportive relationships and safe environments where practitioners are encouraged to reflect critically on their practice, this will assist in the development of individuals capable and confident of practising to best meet the needs of their patients and clients.

Freedom to learn, freedom to be: creating a learning culture

The previous discussions have explored the nature of learning and supporting in practice through the conscious development of adult learning strategies and critical thinking abilities that ensure reflection occurs in and on practice. However, it is essential that we do not rest here as encouraging the idea of the freedom to learn and the freedom to be entails ensuring a suitable environment that sustains the learning individual. The emergence of global markets, rapid information transfer and economic restrictions have hastened calls for the creation of societies and organisations that are more flexible and adaptable in their approach (Barber 1996).

The features of a learning society, as identified by Ball (1992: 384), are that:

◆ learning is accepted as a lifelong activity
◆ learners take personal responsibility for progress
◆ assessment confirms progress not failure
◆ learning is a partnership
◆ capability, personal and shared values, and team working are recognised equally with the pursuit of knowledge.

These are sensible features if learning is to be valued but there also have to be sound economic strategies that support such developments and organisational climates that encourage individual involvement. If the need is for individuals to engage in lifelong learning then it also appears to be a sensible approach to develop the notion of the learning organisation. This entails embracing the characteristics and principles that promote learning from experience and encourage adult learning and the growth of critically reflective employees.

The idea of the learning organisation is not a new one. Argyris and Schon (1978) and Schon (1994) characterised the culture of a learning organisation as one where there was a willingness to experiment and try out new ideas, supported by reflective practice and a keenness to gain insight from experience. This is supported by Handy (1984), who considered learning organisations as those that promised curiosity, discovery and exploration. Sadler (1989) further suggests that a learning organisation must operate within a climate that is open and tolerant in encouraging both creativity and individual respect. A learning organisation then is one that is capable of learning to learn, provides a suitable supportive environment whereby all individuals are involved in learning and is continually engaged in transforming itself (Ball 1992). This is more likely to happen if the principles identified by Swieringa & Wierdsma (1992), are adhered to. These principles concern problem orientation, collective learning, conscious learning and multilayered learning, and are laid out in Table 4.2.

Table 4.2 The learning principles of a learning organisation

Term	Definition
Problem orientation	In the learning organisation problems are seen as challenges, as interesting indicators for change and development. The focus moves from what must be learnt to who learns and how learning occurs
Collective learning	In the learning organisation the emphasis is on learning together as a team, with a central involvement of focus on the interactive nature of learning and the involvement of all members of the organisation. This works by creating a culture of mutual cooperation, blurring of role boundaries and increased opportunities for sharing ideas, taking risks and being creative
Conscious learning	This concerns the provision of a creative environment whereby conscious learning occurs through mutual dialogue and collective enquiry, within an atmosphere of trust, support and mutual respect. The focus for this aspect of the learning organisation is that of an exploration of specific issues and a continual sense of discovery
Multilayered learning	In the learning organisation the atmosphere is one of open dialogue facilitating a variety of approaches to learning at all levels of the organisation. This includes recognition of the rules and principles that permit contradictions and paradoxes. The focus is on critical challenge, debate and the nature of enquiry

Reference: Swieringa & Wierdsma (1992)

To sum up, learning organisations:

◆ are environmentally friendly
◆ ensure open dialogue and challenge
◆ encourage adult learners
◆ are willing to develop and change
◆ embrace innovation
◆ thrive on creativity
◆ support individuals.

This cultural identity may not be readily identifiable in today's NHS, particularly in nursing, where in the past the image and stereotypes of vocation and subservience have produced self-generating occupational strategies of mistrust and insecurity (Davies 1976, Dingwall et al 1988, Hudson-Jones 1988). The effect of these strategies is encapsulated in the following wise words of Celia Davies: 'nurses frequently display the dedication and devotion to their work that is the stuff of public image, but they combine this with an uneasy sense of their own oppression and a seeming belief in their inability to tackle some of the fundamentals that would enable nurses to practise as they would wish' (Davies 1995: 13).

The introduction of 'Project 2000' (UKCC 1986) was heralded as a welcome reform of nursing to provide new recruits, more effective education programmes and the advent of the 'knowledgeable doer'. Sadly the project's rapid implementation and apparent reliance on theoretical aspects to the detriment of clinical skills has resulted in recent demands for a rethink of pre-registration programmes to remedy such skill deficiencies. To lay the blame for nurses' current recruitment and retention ills solely on the implementation of educational reforms is to belie the deep morale problems that arose out of the protracted grading exercise and managerial changes producing a climate where nursing leadership was undervalued (Palmer & Wilson 1997). There is also evidence that direct confrontation between the development of managerialism and traditionally held professional values has also played its part (Pollitt 1990, Morley 1995). Interestingly the move of HCP education into the higher education sector and to degree level seems to have been achieved with limited shroud-waving and angst either from within or outside the professions concerned.

In the context of the current health service climate it would appear a sensible policy to develop innovative strategies and provide for appropriate resources that assist practitioners to take responsibility for their own learning, thus recognising practitioners as adult learners who are:

◆ critical thinkers
◆ self-directed
◆ self-aware
◆ able to problem-solve
◆ able to evaluate experiences
◆ able to recognise the need for continual learning.

If we are to embrace reflection in practice fully and seek the appropriate paths of discovery and strategies that achieve this, then it is reasonable to promote a culture in health care that encourages curiosity, experiment and routes of self-discovery. Such a culture should also promote individual respect and open dialogue through recognised frameworks of professional support. Those practitioners working in new clinical roles will be uniquely placed in responsible and respected positions to ensure that their organisations and their colleagues encourage and support learning individuals. This would go some way to laying the foundations for a learning community in their own professions that could eventually assist the NHS to become a learning organisation and one that is highly valued by those who work in it.

This chapter is dedicated to all those who are continually learning in practice and to Arthur Halstead. I have never met Mr Halstead but it was reported by BBC Radio that he had enrolled on a creative writing course. Arthur Halstead is 97 years old.

REFERENCES

Argyris C, Schon D (1978) Organisational learning. Addison-Wesley, London
Atkins S, Murphy K (1993) Reflection: a review of the literature. Journal of Advanced Nursing 18:1188–1192
Ball C (1992) The learning society. Royal Society of Arts Journal May 380–394
Barber M (1996) The learning game. Arguments for an education revolution. Victor Gollancz, London
Barlow S (1991) Impossible dream. Nursing Times 87(1):53–54
Benner P (1984) From novice to expert: excellence and power in clinical nursing practice. Addison-Wesley, California
Bond M, Holland S (1998) Clinical supervision for nurses. Open University, Buckingham
Boud D (ed) (1995) Enhancing learning through self-assessment. Kogan Page, London
Boud D, Keogh R, Walker D (1985) Reflection: turning experience into learning. Kogan Page, London
Boud D, Miller N (1996) Working with experience: animating learning. Routledge, London
British Broadcasting Corporation (BBC) (1999) New patterns at work – new roles. Discussion, The Business Programme, January
Brookfield S D (1987) Developing critical thinkers. Challenging adults to explore alternative ways of thinking and acting. Open University, Milton Keynes
Brown R (1995) Portfolio development and profiling for nurses, 2nd edn. Quay, Salisbury
Butterworth T, Faugier J (1992) Clinical supervision and mentorship in nursing. Chapman Hall, London
Cameron F (1994) Models of specialist practice. In Humphris D (ed) (1994) Clinical Nurse Specialist: issues in practice. Macmillan, London
Clarke R, Croft P (1998) Critical reading for the reflective practitioner. A guide for primary care. Butterworth-Heinemann, Oxford
Clothier C, MacDonald C A, Shaw D A (1994) The Allitt inquiry. HMSO, London
Cox R (1992) Learning theory and professional life. Media and Technology for Human Development 4(4):217–232
Crouch S (1991) Critical incident analysis. Nursing 4(37):30–31
Davies C (1976) Experience of dependency and control in work: the case of nurses. Journal of Advanced Nursing 1:273–282
Davies C (1995) Gender and the professional predicament in nursing. Open University, Buckingham
Davies N (1993) Murder on ward four. Chatto & Windus, London
Department for Education and Employment (DfEE) (1995) Developing students' subject area knowledge and skills in the workplace. DfEE, London
Department for Education and Employment (DfEE) (1996) Lifelong learning – a consultative document. DfEE, The Scottish Office and The Welsh Office, Edinburgh and Cardiff
Department of Health (DoH) (1993) A vision for the future. The nursing, midwifery and health visiting contribution to health and health care. NHS Management Executive, Department of Health, Leeds
Department of Health (DoH) (1999) Making a difference: strengthening the nursing, midwifery and health visiting contribution to health and health care. Department of Health, London

Dewey J (1933) How we think. A restatement of the relation of reflective thinking to the educative process. Heath, London

Dingwall R, Rafferty A M, Webster C (1988) An introduction to the social history of nursing. Routledge, London

Dobson F (1999) Report to the Commons Health and Select Committee. 27 January. Westminster, London.

Durgahee T (1988) Facilitating reflection: from a sage on the stage to a guide on the side. Nursing Education Today 18:158–164

Eraut M (1994) Developing professional knowledge and competence. Faber, London

Fitzgerald M (1994) Theories of reflection for learning. In Palmer A M, Burns S, Bulman C (eds) Reflective practice in nursing: the growth of the reflective practitioner. Blackwell Science, Oxford

Flanagan J C (1954) The critical incident technique. Psychological Bulletin 51(4):327–358

Foster E (1996) Comparable but different: work-based learning society. The work-based learning project final report 1994–1996. Leeds University and Department for Education and Employment, London

Fowler J, Chevannes M (1998) Evaluating the efficacy of reflective practice within the context of clinical supervision. Journal of Advanced Nursing 27:379–382

Frazer M J (1992) Quality assurance in higher education. Falmer, London

Freire P (1972) Pedagogy of the oppressed. Penguin, London

Gibbs G (1995) Using peer and self-assessment. In Gibbs G Assessing student-centred courses. Oxford Centre for Staff Development, Oxford

Graham I, Waight S, Scammell J (1998) Using structured reflection to improve nursing practice. Nursing Times 94(25):28–31

Greater London Post-Qualifying Education and Training Consortium (GLPQ) (1997) Guidance for candidates on preparation and submission of portfolios. April 1997. GLPQ, London

Handy C (1984) Cited in Goodlad S (ed) Education for the professions. Society for Research into Higher Education and National Foundation for Education Research (NFER)/Nelson, Slough

Hawkins P, Shohet R (1989) Supervision in the helping professions. Open University, Milton Keynes

Horton M (1990) The long haul. Doubleday, New York

Hudson-Jones A (ed) (1988) Images of nurses: perspectives from history, art, literature. University of Pennsylvania, Philadelphia

Hughes L, Pengelly P (1997) Staff supervision in a turbulent environment. Jessica Kingsley, London

Hull C, Redfern L (1996) Profiles and portfolios for nurses and midwives. Macmillan, London

Humphris D (1994) (ed) The clinical nurse specialist: issues in practice. Macmillan, Basingstoke

Jasper M A (1998) Using portfolios to advance practice. In Rolfe G, Fulbrook P (eds) Advanced nursing practice. Butterworth-Heinemann, Oxford

Johns C (1993) Professional supervision. Journal of Nursing Management 1:9–18

Johns C (1998) Opening the doors of perception. In Johns & Freshwater (1998)

Johns C, Freshwater D (1998) Transforming nursing through reflective practice. Blackwell Science, Oxford

Knowles M S (1975) Self-directed learning. Follett, Chicago

Knowles M S (1978) The adult learner: a neglected species, 2nd edn. Gulf, Houston

Kolb D A (1984) Experiential learning. Prentice Hall, New Jersey

Marrow C E, Macauley D M, Crumbie A (1997) Promoting reflective practice through structured clinical supervision. Journal of Nursing Management 5:77–82

Marsick V J, Watkins K (1990) Informal and incidental learning in the workplace. Routledge, London

Miller N, Boud D (1996) Animating learning from experience. In Boud D, Miller N Working with experience. Animating learning. Routledge, London

Morle K M F (1990) Mentorship: is it a case of the emperor's new clothes or a rose by any other name? Nurse Education Today 10(1):66–69

Morley L (1995) Theorising empowerment in the UK public services. Empowerment in Organisations 3(3):35–41

Morton-Cooper A (1998) Preceptorship as transitional learning support: the effects of enablers on adult role learning. Doctoral thesis. Continuing Education Centre, University of Warwick

Morton-Cooper A, Palmer A (1993) Mentoring and preceptorship. A guide to support roles in clinical practice. Blackwell Scientific, Oxford

Morton-Cooper A, Palmer A (2000) Mentoring, preceptorship and clinical supervision. A guide to professional support roles in practice, 2nd edn. Blackwell Science, Oxford

Nicklin P (1995) Super supervision. Nursing Management 2(5):24–25

Palmer A (1987) The nature of the mentor relationship in nurse education. A study to introduce the mentor. Unpublished thesis. South Bank Polytechnic

Palmer A (1996) The learning handbook. The educational package to meet the changing educational needs of midwives in developing new dimensions in care in a variety of settings. English National Board (ENB) & University of Greenwich, London

Palmer A M, Burns S, Bulman C (1994) Reflective practice in nursing: the growth of the reflective practitioner. Blackwell Science, Oxford

Palmer A, Wilson A (1997) New deal: new directions – the evaluation of 'Innovations in practice projects'. South Thames NHS Executive, London

Parsloe E (1995) Coaching, mentoring and assessing. A practical guide to developing competencies, revised edn. Kogan Page, London

Pietroni R, Palmer A (1995) Portfolio-based learning and the role of mentors. Education for General Practice 6:111–114

Pollitt C (1990) Managerialism and the public services: the Anglo-American experience. Blackwell, Oxford

Procter B (1986) A cooperative exercise in accountability. In Marken M, Payne M (eds) Enabling and ensuring. Council for Education and Training in Youth and Community Work, London

Puetz B E (1985) Learn the ropes from a mentor. Nursing Success Today 2(6):11–13

Ramsden P (1992) Learning to teach in higher education. Routledge, London

Redfern L, Roy S (1998) Supervision for nurse specialists. Nursing Times – Learning Curve 2(5):12–13

Roche G R (1979) Much ado about mentors. Harvard Business Review 56, Jan/Feb, 14–28

Rogers C R (1969) Freedom to learn. Charles E Merrill, Columbus, Ohio

Rolfe G (1998) Beyond expertise: reflective and reflexive nursing practice. In Johns C, Freshwater D (eds) Transforming nursing through reflective practice. Blackwell Science, Oxford

Rolfe G, Fulbrook P (1998) (eds) Advanced nursing practice. Butterworth-Heinemann, Oxford

Sadler P (1989) Management development. In Sissons K (ed) Personnel management in Britain. Blackwell, London

Schön D A (1983) The reflective practitioner: how professionals think in action. Basic Books, New York

Schön D (1994) Organisational learning: the core issues. Conference paper presented at the Office for Public Management, London 9–15

Simosko S (1991) APL: a practical guide for professionals. Kogan Page, London

Standing Committee on Postgraduate Medical and Dental Education (SCOPME) (1998) An enquiry into mentoring. Supporting Doctors and Nurses at Work. October 1998. SCOPME, London

Swieringa J, Wierdsma A (1992) Becoming a learning organisation – beyond the learning curve. Addison-Wesley, Wokingham

United Kingdom Central Council for Nursing, Midwifery and Health Visiting (UKCC) (1986) Project 2000: a new preparation for practice. UKCC, London

United Kingdom Central Council for Nursing, Midwifery and Health Visiting

(UKCC) (1996) Position statement on clinical supervision for nursing and health visiting. UKCC, London

United Kingdom Central Council for Nursing, Midwifery and Health Visiting (UKCC) (1998) A higher level of practice. The UKCC's proposals for recognising a higher level of practice within the post-registration regulatory framework. Consultation document. UKCC, London

Van Menen M (1990) The tact of teaching: the meaning of pedagogical thoughtfulness. New York Press, New York

Weil S (1997) Postgraduate education and lifelong learning as collaborative inquiry in action – an emergent model. In Burgess R (ed) Beyond the first degree. Society for Research into Higher Education (SRHE)/Open University (OU) Buckingham

Weil S (1998) Rhetorics and realities in public service organisations: systematic practice and organisational learning as critically reflexive action research (CRAR). Systematic Practice and Action Research 11(1):37–61

Wilson A, Palmer A (1998) Making clinical supervision work: the evaluation report (unpublished). Harrow & Hillingdon Healthcare NHS Trust, Middlesex

FURTHER READING

The following texts are chosen to supplement the references in the chapter as interesting and thought-provoking texts which will further illuminate the experience of learning, reflecting and supporting in practice.

Abbott P, Meerabeau L (1998) The sociology of the caring professions, 2nd edn. University College, London

Capra F (1997) The web of life. A new synthesis of mind and matter. HarperCollins, London

Lawrence G (1983) People types and tiger stripes. A practical guide to learning styles, 2nd edn. Centre for Applications of Psychological Type, Florida

McGrowther J (1995) Profiles, portfolios and how to build them. Scutari, London

Obholzer A, Roberts V Z (eds) The unconscious at work. Routledge, London

Open University (1998) Clinical supervision: a development pack for nurses. School of Health and Social Welfare, Open University, Milton Keynes

Rich A, Parker D (1995) Reflection and critical incident analysis: ethical and moral implications of their use within nursing and midwifery education. Journal of Advanced Nursing 22:1050–1057

Rolfe G (1998) Expanding nursing knowledge. Understanding and researching your own practice. Butterworth-Heinemann, Oxford

Skolimowski H (1994) The participatory mind. A new theory of knowledge and the universe. Penguin, London

5

Managing new roles within the service

Geraldine Walters

Introduction

The subject of management in relation to specialist practice can be viewed from two perspectives; one considers the challenges of managing services against a backdrop of changing clinical roles. The second is concerned with how practitioners with specialist skills can contribute to the management of services they provide. This chapter concentrates predominantly on the situation in nursing, since the issues surrounding specialist practice are particularly marked in nursing and have been well explored. Nevertheless, many of the models of practice suggested, difficulties encountered, and lessons learned apply equally to other non-medical health-care professions (HCPs).

The chapter will also touch upon the recent nurse consultant initiative, which challenges managers to review and negotiate roles and functions to find new and better ways of delivering services. Other HCPs will be interested in the way this development unfolds, since consultant roles in these professions might be developed in the future.

Given the well-documented confusion over titles, in this chapter, for simplicity, the term 'specialist practitioner' encompasses all roles, however titled, which involve any level of 'advanced' clinical practice. The term 'manager' applies to managers with or without clinical backgrounds. By necessity, this chapter will touch upon issues that are explored in greater depth elsewhere in the text.

The views expressed here are personal, and are therefore intended to provoke thought and discussion rather than provide vital and objective data for your next examination or assignment! My impression of where we are, and where we should go in the future in relation to specialist practice has been moulded by my own clinical and managerial nursing experience. This has been in acute NHS settings and in particular, the specialist cardiothoracic environment. Views from other settings may be very different, and it's worth seeking them out.

Background

For nurses who sought greater autonomy and professional influence prior to the 1990s, the NHS reforms of 1989 (Department of Health 1989), the 'New Deal' for Junior Doctors (NHSE 1992), and the 'Scope of Professional Practice'

(UKCC 1992) seemed to herald the sort of opportunities we had all been waiting for. Now, major advances have been made in developing and advancing nursing practice, which are believed to have benefited patients, nurses and their non-nursing colleagues, but much potential remains untapped.

The existence of unexploited potential is anathema in the current, highly pressurised NHS. The difficulties of financing a service fit for the 21st century, the declining popularity of careers in the Health Service (particularly nursing), and recent concerns over clinical quality are resulting in an increasing lack of public confidence. Given such a difficult set of circumstances, it is hard to believe that the skills of nurses and HCPs cannot be better utilised to offer solutions to some of these problems.

Capitalising on the nurse specialist resource in the future will depend upon the development of a robust infrastructure in which the full potential of nurses and HCPs can be achieved, and the ability of professionals themselves to align personal objectives and the objectives of the profession with those of the service. Those in specialist and managerial roles must continue to develop political and organisational awareness to maximise their influence locally and nationally. Evaluation of new roles must also take place to demonstrate how specialist roles can meet the needs of the system and the individuals within it.

This chapter will explore these issues, and is structured as follows:

◆ *The evolution of specialist roles* – this section briefly summarises the evolution of specialist roles, and concentrates on factors which have driven their development, to put this chapter into context
◆ *Infrastructure* – disscusses the infrastructure required to develop specialist practice effectively in order to capitalise on current opportunities, and discusses the inherent difficulties
◆ *Opportunities* – consideration of the opportunities and potential of specialist practice in the NHS today
◆ *Potential models of specialist practice* – gives examples of some models of specialist practice which have been suggested or implemented
◆ *Implementation* – considers the constraints within the system which will impede the development of specialist practice, and suggests the types of change which may be required to overcome these
◆ *Summary and Conclusion.*

The evolution of specialist roles

Groups who have had, and will continue to have, an influence over the way specialist roles evolve are many. These include nurses themselves, nurse and general managers, medical staff, educationalists and professional bodies, and the objectives of these different groups vary. Within individual NHS organisations, specialist role development has often occurred in response to immediate clinical or organisational needs, and consequently implementation has been too rapid to allow the accompanying regulatory and educational foundations to be laid down in advance. Those nurse specialist initiatives that have been led by professional or educational bodies have not always been sufficiently closely aligned to the needs of the service to be successful in practice. It is therefore not surprising that development has been piecemeal and the current situation, although rife with examples of specialist practitioners providing both an excellent and cost-effective service to patients, can best be described as muddled.

In general in nursing, posts which involve a higher level of practice have emerged as a result of one of three types of initiative, nurse specialist developments, nurse practitioner developments, or role expansion in response to the Scope of Professional Practice (UKCC 1992) and the New Deal for Junior Doctors (NHSE 1992). These developments are briefly explained below.

Nurse specialists

Nurse specialists were introduced in the United Kingdom about 20 years ago and their numbers have grown considerably since then. Initially posts such as stoma nurses, continence advisers and diabetic nurse specialists arose out of an appreciation that some patients had specific needs that were not being met by existing medical and nursing staff. The initiative for these posts usually came from the clinical staff delivering the service. They achieved a reduction in medical staff workload and an improvement in the clinical autonomy of nurses, and were also perceived to improve patient care. Posts were not extensively researched or evaluated in the early days of nurse specialism (Humphris 1994). There appears to have been little need to do so – nurses and their medical colleagues were convinced of the benefits of nurse specialists by their own personal experience alone, and this was sufficient to promote an increase in the numbers and types of nurse specialists.

The Royal College of Nursing (RCN) saw the growing demand for specialist nurses as a way to enhance professionalisation and improve career prospects. The RCN envisaged that specialism in nursing should reflect the trend toward greater specialism in medicine and that developments in nursing care would compliment medical advances. In reality, this implementation of the Salmon Report (Ministry of Health 1966) resulted in administrative roles for senior nurses, and the envisaged clinical career structures failed to become a reality.

Nurse practitioners

The nurse practitioner role was originally characterised by being more closely linked to medical practice and the adoption of medical tasks, rather than representing a higher level of 'nurisng'. The role tended to be more generic than the specialty-focused clinical nurse specialists (CNS), and initially practitioners were more common in primary care than in hospital settings. Barbara Stilwell's work (Stilwell 1985) demonstrated that there were value added nursing aspects to nurse practitioner roles, as well as the medical substitution elements. Nurse practitioners are now more common in specialist as well as more generic settings. In the United States, there remains a more distinct demarcation between CNSs and nurse practitioners. CNSs are seen as having a more respectable image among nurse educators, while nurse practitioners are more widely recognised by consumers and other health-care professionals as a good quality but less expensive alternative to doctors (Dunn 1997). In the United Kingdom, the use of nurse practitioners to improve access to primary care for minority groups is being seen as a valuable use of the role (Touche Ross 1994).

After 1990 – 'expanded roles'

The development of so-called 'expanded roles' further complicated the issue of specialist practice. With the advent of the NHS reforms (Department of Health 1989) and the New Deal for Junior Doctors (NHSE 1992), there were different incentives to develop nursing roles incorporating a higher level of practice, but the drive came from managers rather than from clinical staff. The need to reduce junior doctors' hours, and address skill mix and staffing costs to meet the economic objectives of the reformed NHS resulted in scrutiny of medical, nursing and HCP roles and a recommended reallocation of tasks between doctors, nurses, HCPs and untrained support staff. Many of the resulting posts were bestowed with 'practitioner' or 'specialist' titles, regardless of role type or function. Some nurses viewed the simultaneous release of the UKCC standard on the Scope of Professional Practice (UKCC 1992) with suspicion. The desire to expand the nursing role, skills and clinical autonomy was overtaken in some cases by the indignation of being allocated tasks deemed to be inappropriate for junior doctors. Similarly the shifting of some elements of the nursing role to untrained staff was seen as a devaluation of nursing. This was unfortunate, because the opportunities presented for nurses by this initiative were substantial, even if at that point, role expansion was often not accompanied by the status or pay attributed to the clinical nurse specialist, and was more task oriented in nature.

Funding for new nursing and HCP roles was often based on short-term project grants in response to policy changes or acute need, and consequently posts were usually developed at short notice. This rendered many of the posts relatively insecure, not amenable to long-term development or substantial educational preparation for prospective post holders, and rarely part of a long-term human resource strategy. Furthermore, these developments added to the confusion over the definition of the nurse specialist.

Current situation

A view of the current situation regarding new nursing roles in England is provided in a study by McGee et al (1996) and the Department of Health funded 'Exploring new roles in practice' (ENRiP) study (School of Health and Related Research 1999). Not surprisingly, the trends in the findings of both studies were similar. The ENRiP study was carried out between 1996 and 1997, and identified 603 nursing and 235 HCP posts in a 20% sample of Trusts in England, described by their organisations as new roles in practice. Of the nursing roles, 33% had 'specialist' in the job title, and 16% had 'practitioner' while 51% had other titles. Differences in title seemed to boil down to preference of one particular title over another rather than an attempt to describe the post based on the content of the role. Titles of the HCP roles were not analysed because they tended to reflect the postholder's grade in managerial terms or seniority (e.g. Superintendent or Senior 1) rather than giving any indication as to the specialist nature of their work. Educational preparation was inconsistent. McGee et al similarly found no standard job descriptions for specialist practitioner roles, even within the same organisation. They also attempted to identify the differences between 'specialist' and 'advanced' practitioners in terms of scope of practice, but found little differentiation between the two.

The ad hoc nature of role development has advantages and disadvantages as far as development of specialist practice in the future is concerned. A major disadvantage seems to be that the resulting mix of roles will be difficult to handle when considering the crucial questions of defining, regulating and developing roles in the future. Advantages are that these were the pioneering roles and some have succeeded in demonstrating the skill and ability of nurses and HCPs to those who may have previously been unsupportive of such professionals practising in a clinically autonomous fashion. The experiences of postholders and the longer-term sustainability of these roles will also help identify more precisely the successful models for new clinical role development in the future.

Infrastructure

The current confusion in terms of roles and functions has resulted from there being no nationally recognised infrastructure to support the development of specialist practice, and is major limitation for anyone involved in its development. Without such an infrastructure, from the managers' point of veiw, there are concerns over roles and responsibilities, accountability and liability. From the professionals' point of view accountability is also an issue, as are issues concerned with marketability and transferability of skills and experience, remuneration and career planning.

Components of the infrastructure

An infrastructure to support specialist practice should encompass the following:

◆ Regulation and role definition
◆ Education
◆ Career development and remuneration
◆ Evaluation.

Establishing these components is complex. The purpose of regulation is to safeguard patients, and allows the setting and audit of standards to assure of safe practice. It also provides employers with a framework regarding the employment and role of practitioners, and makes the role more understandable to the public and to other health-care professionals. However, before decisions regarding regulation, education and remuneration can take place, the service must define what it requires of specialists in order to specify the role. The problem is therefore somewhat 'chicken and egg' in nature, and is further hampered by the understandable unwillingness of the service to invest in new roles before the benefits to patients have been demonstrated. It is, therefore, not surprising that elements of the infrastructure are not properly in place, and that similar problems in developing and recognising specialist roles are common in many countries where there are organised health-care systems.

Development of local infrastructures

In the absence of a nationally defined infrastructure, some individual Trusts are attempting to formulate their own infrastructures to assist in the systematic development of specialist practice at local level. An effective infrastructure at individual Trust level should at least ensure that definition of specialist roles, pay scales and reporting relationships are consistent across the organisation, and that standards for educational preparation, supervision and audit are in place.

A drawback is that development of a worthwhile local infrastructure requires a lot of time and effort which some are unwilling to commit when a national infrastructure may emerge at a later date. This could also potentially result in the need for re-accreditation or retraining of people in whom an investment in training has already been made. Secondly, a proliferation of different local infrastructures results in variations between different organisations in education, standards of practice and role definition. From the point of view of the nurse, skills and status are less transferable (although this may appeal to managers who are aiming to retain skilled nursing staff!). One could also argue that the current fragmented situation regarding specialist practitioners is the result of differing local developments in the past.

However, since the concept of specialist practice is now better understood, a well-developed local infrastructure is probably a risk worth taking, and is one which many Trusts are attemping in a more systematic way than previously. The disadvantages of developing a local infrastructure are minimised if local organisations collaborate to achieve some consistency within the same geographical area. Achieving some basic agreements between separate organisations within the education consortium would also increase the momentum to commission specific educational programmes to support specialist practice.

The following sections will discuss the individual components of this infrastructure, whether locally or nationally formulated.

Role definition

It is crucial that definition of the role is agreed as a baseline from which to specify educational, remunerative and regulatory criteria. This section will focus on definitions applied to specialist practice in nursing.

The majority of definitions of nurse specialists to date have originated from the professional bodies, some examples from the UK and USA are shown in Box 5.1.

Professional – service tensions

The definitions shown in Box 5.2 tend to reflect Hamric's primary criteria for the nurse specialist, which include expert practitioner, educator, researcher and consultant (Hamric 1989). The definitions suggest an all-encompassing role, although CNS and nurse practitioner roles in the UK have not traditionally incorporated this range of activities (Manley 1993). In the US, CNS roles are more likely to incorporate these elements in theory, although research has shown that this may not be the case in practice. To give an example, clinical nurse specialists spend less than 3% of their time involved in research activities during the first two years following qualification (Cooper and Sparacino 1990, cited in Woods 1998).

In practice, roles tend to be shaped by the needs and pressures of the service, rather than the definitions formulated from within the profession. When service pressures come into play, tensions arise (see Box 5.2).

Box 5.1 Definitions of specialist practice

◆ Specialist practice involves a clinical and consultative role, teaching, management, research and the application of relevant nursing research. Only if a nurse is involved in all of these is he or she a specialist (RCN 1988).

◆ Nurses in advanced clinical practice have a graduate degree in Nursing. They conduct comprehensive health assessments and demonstrate a high level of autonomy and expert skill in the diagnosis of complex responses of individuals, families and communities to actual or potential health problems. They formulate clinical decisions to manage acute and chronic illness and promote wellness. Nurses in advanced clinical practice integrate education, research, management leadership and consultation into their clinical role. They function in collegial relationships with nursing peers, physicians, professionals and others who influence the health environment (*American Nurses' Association Congress of Nursing Practice, cited in McLoughlin 1992*).

◆ A nurse prepared beyond the level of nurse generalist and authorised to practice as a specialist with advanced clinical expertise in the nursing field. Specialist experience to ensure competency in speciality practice includes clinical, teaching, administration, research and consultant roles. Post-basic education for speciality practice is a formally recognised programme of study built upon the general education for the nurse and providing the content and experience to ensure competency in speciality practice (*International Council of Nurses 1992*).

Box 5.2 Professional – service tension

Woods (1998) carried out a study to look at factors which appeared to promote or limit the development of specialist roles, using a cohort of students undertaking a Masters degree preparation. Factors associated with re-negotiating relationships and adapting to becoming a nurse specialist were identified as important, and issues surrounding the deployment and environment in which practitioners worked were also identified. The most common factor cited in relation to the latter point was that some of the practitioners were not supernumerary within their clinical areas, and therefore sickness and lack of resources would often result in the abandonment of the advanced practice role to manage and supervise the clinical area.

For a manager of a service, the retention of an additional skilled member of staff to call upon during times of heavy workload or staff shortage may be sufficiently attractive to justify the investment in the training and establishment of an specialist practitioner post. However, the practitioners in this study identified this situation as severely limiting to the development of the role.

The difficulties in aligning the practical reality with the definitions of the professional bodies probably stem from the lack of any service-led definitions of specialist roles, incorporating the objectives of non-clinical managers or patients. The aspirations of the two are likely to be different. For example, the nursing definitions reflect a longer-term perspective of the type of role that nurses aspire to, which would improve the professional status of nursing, and would provide the care that they believe would be in the best interests of patients. Managers' views are more influenced by the financial pressures of today, in delivering health services in a climate of decreasing budgets and increasing user expectations, and are looking for a service that will provide an immediate solution to some of these problems. Their priorities are therefore to fulfil service needs and increase quality, but without an increase, and preferably with a reduction, in cost. Increasing the professional status of nursing is less important to the non–nurse manager.

The manager's viewpoint is not difficult to understand. In the short term, 'true' specialist posts are relatively expensive in terms of salary costs, training and development requirements, and supervision. Many of the perceived cost benefits of specialist posts arise in the longer term, from added value in terms of higher quality care, shorter lengths of stay, fewer re-admissions, better patient compliance with treatment, fewer complaints and, possibly, less litigation. These benefits are not easily quantifiable when formulating a business case to support a specialist post, and the 'pay back' for investment in specialists cannot be recouped in the short term. The need for directorates to break even annually, sometimes on a fairly small budget, limits the ease with which specialist posts can be developed. Similarly, although the development of specialist practice as a means of improving the status of the profession to positively impact recruitment and retention in the longer term is currently a popular idea, the speed, and even the likelihood of success, of this strategy cannot be predicted.

It is therefore important that service and professional requirements are both taken into consideration when defining the role of the nurse specialist in local infrastructure development. In nursing, the Nurse Director should have an understanding and a commitment to both professional and service requirements and is theoretically in a key position to reconcile the needs of both in developing a nurse specialist role. To do this effectively, Nurse Directors' appreciate the need to adopt an approach that is sensitive to the operational management constraints of clinical directorates without compromising professional development.

To take an extreme example, the Nurse Director may be presented with the desire to create a nurse specialist post which is under-funded, poorly supervised, or offers little in the way of specialised practice as it is defined by the profession, as an economical solution to a service problem. A supportive and pragmatic approach to find solutions to the problem is required, by assessing service needs, establishing how these may be met and whether a nurse specialist role is actually what is required. Specialist posts that are conceptually acceptable but inadequately funded in terms of salary provision may still be practical if there is agreement to review pay scales after evaluation of the post. This may also be feasible if it is likely that a postholder will need further education and development in order to fulfil the role. Recognition of the necessity for supervision or audit of practice is enshrined in new clinical governance arrangements, and convincing managers of the necessity for adequate arrangements in this regard should now be easier.

Intra-professional tension

In addition to the disparity that sometimes exists between nurses and managers over what should constitute specialist role, in nursing in particular, there is also a level of disagreement within the profession in relation to the appropriateness of different types of tasks and their allocation which must be resolved. There is reluctance by some nurses to delegate some of the tasks which have historically been 'core' to the nursing role, to untrained staff, and to adopt tasks which have been within in the scope of practice of medical staff. This former point reflects the view that provision of basic care is more associated with caring and nurturing than are tasks such as examining patients, ordering and administering treatment, or undertaking complex monitoring of vital signs. Nursing must resolve such arguments, which are internal to the profession, in order to develop a unified approach to professional development that is in line with the needs of the service and of patients.

A personal argument, as a nurse and a manager, is that 'caring' can be associated with any physical task being undertaken, what really matters is the approach, skill and sensitivity of the person who is undertaking it. It is acknowledged that skills are required to provide basic care for patients. Although tasks such as bathing or feeding patients are technically basic, both activities are good opportunities to interact with the patient, assess, identify, treat and therefore avoid potential problems. That only individuals who have undergone nurse training and have nursing experience can possess these skills is unlikely, although supervision by a trained nurse, if unqualified individuals were performing these tasks, would be preferable. The ability of nurses to provide care and comfort for patients is more likely to be impeded by the current tensions within the role, generated by the growing need to adopt more technical tasks in addition to the basic care requirements. Health care is becoming increasingly technical and this has implications for the nursing role. Nursing therefore needs to evolve in the same direction in order to continue to meet changing patient needs, embracing new roles and being prepared to divest itself of those which can be safely delegated with supervision. Nurturing and caring do not need to be sacrificed in order to do this.

Education

There is little disagreement in the belief that specific post-registration educational preparation is required to function as a specialist in any health-care profession. There are questions over what that preparation should consist of and at what academic level. In the UK, the principle of graduate-level entry for specialist nurses was stated by the UKCC in 1994 as a requirement within the standards for PREP (UKCC 1994), but the issue over whether graduate-level preparation is required for basic registration results in confusion. If some newly qualified nurses are graduates, what level of educational preparation would they require to become a nurse specialist?

In the US, to overcome the difficulties of different job titles and levels of educational preparation of nurses working in specialist practitioner roles, the solution has been to create a further level, entitled 'advanced practice', requiring Masters level education. This would potentially include all those practitioners functioning in specialist roles, either as nurse practitioners or clinical specialists. The justification for this is that a higher level of graduate entry will improve the credibility of nurses working at this level in the eyes of other health-care workers.

The UKCC has not agreed an educational framework for advanced practice. Manley's experience in implementing an advanced practitioner role according to Hamric's definition suggested that there is a need for education and practical experience in all aspects of the role, i.e. educator, consultant and researcher (Manley 1997), a guarantee that post-holders will have the skills to undertake research and teaching components of their role. For nurse specialists of the future to fulfil a more corporate, strategic role effectively, there is also an argument for more educational preparation in health service management, finance and planning (see Box 5.3).

Box 5.3 Business awareness

'Concerns about cost and financial accountability are not the sole responsibility of the nurse manager or administrator.... To be effective, CNSs must learn to speak the language of business along with the language of clinical patient care. A collaborative approach between manager and clinician is essential to establish quality patient services at an economical cost to the organisation. The timely facilitation of the integration of financial acumen will establish the CNS as an invaluable resource in health care planning' (Boyle 1997).

The increasing level and scope of formal and theoretical education being recommended for specialist practitioner is sure to cause some concern within the profession. To give an indication of the level of educational preparation being suggested, Manley recommends preparation at Doctoral level to assure competence in research (Manley 1997). Nursing has a substantial practical element and although graduate status may contribute to professionalisation, and a sound knowledge base is undoubtedly required, practitioners whose strengths lie primarily in their practical skills and compassion may be disadvantaged or lost to the profession. There is, therefore, a need to develop robust methods of assessing and accrediting practical competence to contribute towards the acquisition of a degree. This will ensure that the maximum number of competent practitioners can achieve the award, and conversely ensure that knowledge is accompanied by sound practical skills.

Career structures

Career development is a particular problem for specialists. Nurses specialist roles have traditionally focused on a narrow clinical field. Once competence has been reached, there is a risk of specialists suffering a degree of boredom in repeatedly dealing with the same types of clinical issues. The prospects for increasing salary or developing their careers further in the health service are limited without moving back into mainstream practice (often a downward or sideways step), usually to find a route into management. To ensure that clinical specialists remain motivated and challenged, development of the co-ordinating, managerial, research or educative elements of specialist practitioner roles as suggested in most of the definitions would seem sensible. While this would be a useful development, the extent of direct patient contact for the nurse specialist would be reduced. The fact that many specialist practitioners chose a specialist clinical career because they sought a more autonomous clinical role and wished to retain patient contact therefore presents a problem. This option also risks invitation of the familiar criticism, that skilled clinical nurses are disincentivised from remaining in the clinical area by lack of opportunities for career development, and instead are 'lost' to patient care by moving into more administrative roles.

This conundrum is a very difficult one, possibly because we are seeking a solution to an insoluble problem. In practically every profession, the more senior roles become, the greater the administrative and managerial component of the role. The challenge is therefore to retain the clinical focus of the role of the specialist nurse (possibly by the nurse specialist maintaining a small case load), but to incorporate elements of management, research and education, and enhance the status of nurse specialists to ensure that their input is actively sought when strategic decisions are made. This essentially mirrors the role of the medical consultant. The key question is, therefore, whether this status can be awarded to nurse specialists, or whether the nurse specialists themselves need to develop strategies to achieve it. It is probably a combination of both and is very dependent on the culture and nature of the organisations in which nurse specialists work, and the aspirations and drive of the nurse specialists themselves (see Box 5.4). Recent opportunities will assist in the enhancement of the status of nursing, provided these are fully exploited by nurses themselves.

Box 5.4 Clinical specialist longevity

Boyle (1997) carried out a qualitative study among a small sample of clinical nurse specialists in the US who had held posts for more than 10 years, to identify which factors had contributed to their career longevity. Several key organisational factors were important, primarily:

◆ the nurse having an advocate at senior administrative level (usually the Director of Nursing) who supports and sponsors them

◆ having a similar clinical supporter and mentor (usually a medical consultant)

◆ a vibrant organisation, offering variety and change and a degree of freedom and independence.

Other factors were personal to the CNSs themselves. Long serving CNSs were often proactive individuals who sought to publicise and market their own roles within and outside the organisation. They felt that they had found their niche in clinical practice, were proud of their contribution to patients, to the development of junior nurses, and the service. In other words, there was a level of fit between what the organisation required of them, and what they required from their role.

Remuneration

The current situation regarding remuneration reflects the confusion over titles, roles and educational preparation, with no consistency in the grading of nurse specialist posts (McGee et al 1996). In McGee's study, 'Specialist' nurses graded between D and I were identified. It is likely that the more extreme differences in pay result from anomalies in job titles rather than a lack of parity between individuals who are fulfiling similar roles. What an appropriate remuneration strategy for nurse specialists may be is more difficult problem.

Nurses' pay has always been high on the agenda within the profession. The issue is becoming a more urgent problem for the Government in the light of the current recruitment and retention difficulties in nursing. The root of the current recruitment crisis is multifactorial, incorporating pay, status, working conditions, lack of a clinical career structure, and confusion over whether nursing is a graduate profession or not to the potential recruit. Some change is required to ensure that the service can be manned in the future. Nurse specialism, and the new concept of nurse consultants is being regarded as a tool to aid recruitment and retention using the prospect of higher status and pay offered by these roles.

If nursing does become increasingly specialist in nature, requiring educational preparation at first degree or Master level, then the terms and conditions offered must be commensurate with other graduate-based careers that are open to potential recruits. There must also be sufficient numbers of these 'higher pay, higher status' roles within the system to offer this particular opportunity to the majority of new recruits if this strategy is to be successful. This would result in an additional large tier of highly paid nurses, relative to the current situation. There would undoubtedly be benefits, but could the Health Service afford it? Again, the answer could be yes, provided the introduction of greater numbers of nurse specialists results in demonstrable cost savings and as well as benefits in terms of quality.

Evaluation

Given the above argument, evaluation of posts is crucial to demonstrate the cost and quality benefits to the service, otherwise it is difficult to justify additional investment in specialist practitioners, and set a level of remuneration which is affordable and appropriate.

Evaluation of the value of nursing has been a problem for the profession. Firstly, nursing is a relatively new profession in the academic sense and consequently research is in its infancy. Secondly, the precise contribution of nursing to patient care and outcome is notoriously difficult to tease out because nursing input is a constant feature throughout a patient's health care experience, and is inextricably linked with a host of other influences. For these reasons, and perhaps also as a result of preference within the profession, nursing is more amenable to study using qualitative research methods. Such methods cannot be easily applied to economic evaluation, and have historically not been acknowledged by the medical profession, who favour a positivist, quantitative approach. The majority of work that has demonstrated benefits of specialist practitioners has involved those working with narrow client groups and those who have a specific caseload, although there has been little analysis of cost benefits (Wilson-Barnett 1995). It is easier to exclude other influences in these situations, and consequently the individual input of the specialist practitioner is more amenable to evaluation.

In spite of these limitations, research into specialist practice is becoming more achievable. Qualitative research is becoming more universally accepted in health care. The emphasis on health services research generally is increasing with the advent of the NHS Central Research and Development Strategy and the clinical effectiveness and evidence-based practice initiatives. The need to undertake research or audit is now a more common feature within nursing job descriptions, particularly those that involve a higher level of practice. The increase in graduate-level education in nursing has meant that increasing numbers of nurses have been exposed to, and have had some experience in, the practice of research. It is hopeful, then, that having gained the ability to evaluate nursing developments in a robust and scientific fashion, a better case for investment in specialist nurses can be made. Evaluation of specialist roles needs to begin now, and specialist nurses themselves should take the initiative. Box 5.5 provides some guidelines.

Box 5.5 Evaluating specialist roles

Specialist nurses may wonder where to begin with their research. Suggested guidelines are:

◆ Find out what sort of things your organisation is interested to know.

◆ Who are your advocates at a senior level?

◆ What evidence do your supporters need to market your role to the Board? Translate their broad ideas into smaller, answerable questions.

◆ Collaborate. Seek some help from experienced researchers in the area you are interested in, either within your organisation or your local education provider.

◆ Explore the possibility of registering for a higher degree with your research. (If you are going to do it any way, why not formalise it?)

◆ Don't expect too much, too soon. Research is usually a long, slow process.

Current opportunities

It is important to streamline the situation with regard to specialist roles. This will enable nurses and HCPs to seize the opportunities offered by recent policy changes outlined in the White Paper, 'The New NHS – Modern, Dependable' (Department of Health 1997a), and help resolve current difficulties in delivering health care, associated with the recruitment and retention crisis across a number of health care professions. Development of nurse consultants will be a key driver for new developments in nursing, and the provision of supporting policy increases the chances of success of the initiative. These issues are discussed below.

'The new NHS – modern, dependable'

'The new NHS – modern, dependable' outlines changes in the organisation of health care, and inherent in this document are new opportunities to formalise the input, and therefore enhance the status, of nursing. The White Paper does not make specific reference to other HCPs, but it seems inevitable that they too are likely to experience continuing pressure to develop new roles.

◆ At primary care level, it is envisaged that new primary care groups consisting of local General Practitioners and community nurses will work together as teams to shape local services. This structure is aimed at aligning clinical and financial responsibility, giving clinical staff the ability to use resources to meet clinical need as they see fit. The input of nurses will formalise the role of experienced clinical nurses in contributing to strategic decisions in primary care.

◆ A new approach toward clinical and service quality is described. Disease-specific service frameworks will be developed to ensure consistency in clinical care across the country. The Calman-Hine Report on Cancer Services (Department of Health 1994) is a pre-existing example of such a framework, which specifies that cancer patients should be cared for by specialist nurses. The precise meaning of this requirement is questionable (i.e., should all care be actually delivered by a nurse with specialist training, or does this just refer to care co-ordination and supervision, and what is the definition of 'specialist' in this sense). The endorsement of specialist nursing and nurse-led services within this framework is an acknowledgement of the importance of skilled nursing in care provision.

Recruitment and retention

A further 'opportunity' of sorts is the recruitment and retention crisis in nursing, which is encouraging the Government and local Trust Executives to look more closely at meeting the needs of nurses locally and nationally, and to address ways of increasing the attraction of nursing as a career. The time is now ripe for nurses and HCPs to make a case specifying what they can offer the service, and outlining what they want in return.

Recent nursing developments

In 1998, the Prime Minister announced the Government's commitment to look into the creation of Nurse Consultant posts (NHSE 1998). The stated aim of the initiative was to give those senior clinical nurses who may otherwise enter management the option of furthering their careers in the clinical field. The posts, it was intended, should be of the same status in nursing as consultant doctors are in medicine. The concept was guardedly welcomed within the profession but there was some cynicism regarding the lack of any mention of nurse consultant pay. The point was also made that creating an elite would not solve the current problems of staff shortage and low nursing pay across the board.

This announcement was followed one year later by three policy documents which progressed the understanding of the role and function of the nurse consultant, and how this new role fits into a proposed new career framework for nurses, midwives and health visitors. The documents were:

◆ The National Nursing, Midwifery and Health Visiting Strategy 'Making a Difference: Strengthening the Nursing, Midwifery and Health Visiting Contribution to Health and Healthcare' (NHSE 1999a)
◆ HSC 1999/217: Nurse, Midwife and Health Visitor Consultants: Establishing New Posts and Making Appointments, appended to which was the UKCC higher level of practice pilot standards (NHSE 1999b)
◆ Advance Letter (NM) 2/1999 Nurse, Midwife and Health Visitor Consultants 1999/2000 (NHSE 1999c).

The nursing strategy 'Making A Difference' provides concrete guidance on a development of a four-stage clinical career pathway from health care assistant/cadet, to registered nurse, nurse specialist, and, finally, nurse consultant. The key elements of the infrastructure for developing practice are incorporated in objectives for professional regulation, education and training, and new roles and skills. The relationship between achievement of the objectives of the White Paper and how the required professional developments in nursing, midwifery and health visiting will be achieved are made explicit.

HSC 1999/217 'Nurse, Midwife and Health Visitor Consultants: Establishing New Posts and Making Appointments' gave guidance about the nature of the nurse consultant role. The guidance makes the specific point that the nurse consultant is a new role – as opposed to a title bestowed on a practitioner working in an existing one, and that the role should be created to meet a defined health need. The guidance also specified that 50% of the post holder's time should be spent in contact with patients. Incorporated in the guidance was the UKCC standard for a higher level of practice (which is likely to lead to regulation of higher level practice in the future). In support of this document, advance letter 2/1999 set out a pay scale for nurse consultants of up to £40,000.

Therefore, after 20 years of ad hoc development of specialist roles, these three documents in a short space of time have established the core of a nationally recognised infrastructure, which has previously been lacking. The publication of tight guidance on the definition, creation and appointment to Nurse Consultant posts, including the requirement for the initial posts to be approved by regional offices of the NHS Executive, reduces the risk of the 'nurse consultant' becoming just another title.

Provision of the national guidance described above simplifies the development of more formal local infrastructures. The challenge for managers is now to manage a process of change, to ensure that new policy is implemented to improve service delivery, introduce (if they choose) the new nurse consultant role and assist staff to identify their position in the new career structure. For some, this change will be difficult. Some nurses with specialist skills will undoubtedly be fulfilling posts that meet the specifications of the nurse consultant guidance while others with similar titles are not. Issues of equity and fairness will arise, and there will be variations in the interpretation and implementation of the initiative nationwide. There are no easy solutions to assure complete equity and fairness, and the task of local managers will be to make sure that nurses are well informed and able to contribute to decision making at individual orgnisational level, and that processes are transparent. An important issue will be to make a clear distiction between the role of the nurse specialist and nurse consultant.

Models for new roles in nursing

Models of specialist practice have previously been suggested which described the specialist nurse as manager/leader, case manager, or fulfilling the more holistic nursing role in the spirit of Hamric's definition. These are described below. With the advent of the nurse consultant role, and the proposed moves to a four-tier clinical career structure, all require some modification, and a decision on where the two roles of specialist and consultant now sit in relation to one another.

Specialist as leader

The UKCC's framework for post-registration education and practice requires entry to specialist practice at graduate level. The model inferred is one of the clinical nurse specialist leading a team of non-specialist nurses, newly qualified clinical specialists, and vocationally trained health-care assistants.

Castledine (1998) suggests a similar model, involving a three-tier structure of nurses headed by a 'senior clinical nurse'. The senior clinical nurse is defined as an individual who has 5-to-10 years' clinical experience, has attained a reasonable academic level, and is respected by colleagues. The prime function of the senior clinical nurse would be to provide clinical leadership for nursing. The role would involve:

◆ improving the quality of nursing care using activities such as practice development, research, standard setting, audit and clinical supervision
◆ some delivery of care and treatment previously regarded as being within the medical domain
◆ practice would extend across the traditional professional, service and agency boundaries, focussing on the provision of holistic health care and promotion of wellness.

The more junior tier of the structure would consist of post-registration general nurses in any of the four general specialities. The middle tier would consist of 'generalist nurse experts' and 'specialist nurse experts'. The model allows nurses to move within and between bands, without financial penalty, to gain expertise, as generalists or specialists. Progress from tier to tier is based on experience, competency and knowledge. Education to degree level would be required to move from the more junior tier to the expert tier, in keeping with PREP requirements. The use of unqualified health-care assistants is not referred to in the Castledine model. The emphasis on working across care and agency boundaries, and the underlying theme of health promotion are very much in keeping with objectives within the Green paper 'Our Healthier Nation' (Department of Health 1997b).

The nurse consultant could fulfil the role of leader in this model, although there is a danger that the administration element of the job will eventually preside during times of heavy workload and staff shortage, and the clinical aspects would be jeopardised as described in the example discussed earlier. The objective for nurse consultants to spend 50% of time in clinical practice would therefore be difficult to achieve. An alternative would be for the nurse consultant to sit 'outside' these frameworks, to be consulted upon as required. However, in this situation, the ability to influence service organisation and management would be lost.

Specialist as case manager

In this case the nurse specialist is attached to a specific group of patients and is involved in evaluation, diagnosis, and treatment. An example from the US is the advanced practice nurse role in surgical services, described by Hylka and Beschle (1997). Advanced practice nurses in this setting are qualified to Masters level. Operationally, an advanced practice nurse and a surgeon are assigned to each patient admitted for a surgical procedure. Both professionals follow the patient throughout their length of stay. This reduces fragmentation of care, improves communication between professionals and between professionals, patients and their family.

The role of the advanced practice nurse in this setting involves:

◆ carrying out all pre-surgical procedures including history taking, requesting and organising tests and investigations, and providing pre-operative information and education
◆ acting as first assistant during the operative procedure
◆ managing post-operative care using protocols
◆ maintaining contact with the patients' family throughout, providing follow-up care and assisting the patient back into the community.

This role integrates all facets of patient education, research, resource management, leadership and staff consultation, and the nurse has a collaborative and equitable relationship with general nurses, medical staff and other health-care professionals. It is easy to envisage how an experienced nurse acting in this capacity could make an impact on continuity of care and communication, and for methodological reasons, this impact would be easier to measure scientifically than the previous models described. It is difficult to envisage how a nurse could further her career clinically beyond this role; therefore the level of remuneration would need to be set at an acceptable level to recruit and retain nurses in such a post. For these reasons, one could envisage the role, with some modification, as being appropriate for a nurse consultant. However, this model is also less conducive to allowing the incumbent to influence strategic development of services unless the job plan was tightly specified. Also, although the authors argue that this is not a technical or medical substitution role, the cynical may disagree. There are also clearly disadvantages for medical staff training and experience, and medical staff training should possibly be a sub-role in order to overcome this.

Hamric's model

Manley (1997) describes an action research project in which the advanced practitioner/nurse consultant role based on Hamric's model and criteria, which reflects the US ideal of advanced nursing, was operationalised in a UK Nursing Development Unit. The developing role involved direct care of patients and their families, working with staff in planning care for their patients and developing evidence-based protocols, supervising staff and guiding them in reflective practice, and exploring practice issues. Manley concluded that in the UK setting, the practical and theoretical skill of the advanced practitioner is of little value without the right context in which to place the role. Three prerequisites were identified for the successful operationalisation, these were:

◆ shared values and beliefs
◆ open and non-hierarchical unit management
◆ organisational authority attributed to the post.

Manley makes the point that nursing development units tend to be established with a culture of shared values and open management and therefore these influences were already strong in the unit in which the work took place. Further research would be needed to ascertain the ease of implementing the model in different settings where this cultural background was not present. Regarding the third point, in the study in question, the researcher did not have a position of power within the organisation. It was recognised that holders of such posts need to be recognised as senior within the organisation, with equal status within the senior nurse management team, and should be an active contributor to the Trust strategy. This element of the role was not operationalised within this particular project, and the need to further describe and demonstrate the effect of such roles on outcomes in order to convince Trust managers, the Government and the public of their value, presumably to promote this status, was emphasised.

Summary

The models described by UK authors tend to lean towards definitions of specialist practice by the professional bodies and encompass the variety of sub-roles suggested by them. In terms of how the nurse consultant may be introduced, since the guidance on the proposed nurse consultant posts is more service orientated, the more specific service related example from the US appears to be a better 'fit'. However, it is difficult to argue the case for a particular model of practice. Individual studies are a useful insight, but do not indicate the ease with which specific models could be applied in practice on a large scale. There is still some way to go in deciding how the new career structure could work in practice.

Implementation

It is likely that models of specialist/consultant practice would need to be modified to suit particular settings. The principles that I believe should be encompassed within an infrastructure for specialist practice are outlined in Box 5.6.

As a manager, I have doubts as to whether specialist practice could be implemented according to these principles affordably, without a shift of money from somewhere else within the Health Service. In nursing, a solution that has been suggested is a reduction in size of the trained workforce.

Box 5.6 Specialist consultant practice – principles

◆ Practice should be regulated.

◆ Preparation should involve Masters-level education and a defined amount of practical experience in the speciality.

◆ The pay structure should be commensurate with other professions requiring Masters-level education.

◆ Clinical career structures should be developed – senior clinical managers of the future should have a specialist background and retain a clinical caseload.

◆ Junior professionals should be en route to specialist/consultant practice within a defined career pathway.

Trained nurses would consist of a smaller group, most of whom would either be specialist/consultant nurses or training to be so. There would be an increase in generic workers who would provide basic care under the supervision of nurse specialists and consultants. The generic worker role would also be a precursor to nurse training for those who opted to enter the profession by that route. This suggestion has been made in various fora and is not a universally popular one. An unfortunate fact is that the pool of trained nurses is already decreasing, but without the commensurate increase in specialist nurses.

To achieve this a total workforce strategy is required which would involve a review of the roles and consequently the education of all professional groups in health care (Box 5.7).

Box 5.7 A strategy for the whole workforce

◆ Developing new roles in practice should be part of a total workforce strategy encompassing all professional groups, including medical staff.

◆ Educational preparation and roles should be spread across professional boundaries and be directly linked to service requirements.

◆ Some linkage of educational funding streams will be required.

Individual organisations do have the ability to develop a workforce strategy along these lines independently, by restructuring establishments and experimenting with different types of roles, responsibilities and pay structures across different staff groups. However, this is a radical approach and requires a large investment in education, training, and staff consultation, which is difficult for organisations to achieve in isolation. Many organisations are naturally reluctant to take this on, particularly in the light of impending national guidelines on job evaluation and pay. Organisation-specific solutions also result in incremental changes only to roles in individual organisations, rather than the radical rethink in the structure of nursing, medicine and other health-related professions, their regulation and their education, which is required. The need for centrally initiated action remains an important one.

Conclusion

This chapter has explored ways in which specialism in nursing and HCPs is being developed to make an impact on the provision of health care in the future. It has considered the background to explain the current situation and suggests the infrastructure required to achieve maximum benefit in the future. In nursing, recent policy initiatives have contributed considerably to the development of this infrastructure. Examples of models of specialist practice have been summarised, and a number of tensions that are at the heart of the development of specialist practice have been examined.

In addition to whatever changes happen nationally or locally, to ensure that nurses and HCPs can contribute meaningfully to the service in the future, they must share the objectives of the system in which they work and be willing to shape new roles accordingly. This requires political and organisational awareness, but is achievable without abandoning the more traditional professional values. Recent changes in Government policy, and the recruitment and retention crisis also offer nurses and HCPs the most profound opportunities there have been for some time to redefine their status, roles and autonomy, both clinical and organisational. The inherent opportunities for the professions and the service should not be missed.

REFERENCES

Boyle D M (1997) Lessons learned from clinical nurse specialist longevity. Journal of Advanced Nursing 26(6):1168–1174
Castledine G (1998) The future of specialist and advanced practie. In Castledine G, McGee P (eds) Advanced and specialist nursing practice. Blackwell Science, Oxford
Department of Health (DoH) (1989) Working for patients. HMSO, London
Department of Health (DoH) (1994) A policy framework for commissioning cancer services ('Calman–Hine report'). HMSO, London
Department of Health (DoH) (1997a) The new NHS: modern, dependable. Stationery Office, London
Department of Health (DoH) (1997b) Our healthier nation – a contract for health. Stationery Office, London
Hamric A (1989) A model for CNS evaluation. In Hamric A, Spross J (eds) The clinical nurse specialist in theory and practice, 2nd edn. W B Saunders, Philadelphia, pp 83–104

Humphris D (ed) (1994) The clinical nurse specialist: issues in practice. Macmillan, Basingstoke

Hylka S C, Beschle J C (1997) The role of advanced practice nurses in surgical services. Association of Operating Room Nurses (AORN) Journal 66(3) September:481–485

International Council for Nurses (1992) Guidelines on specialisation in nursing. R(96) 1. Commission of the European Communities, Brussels

Manley K A (1993) The clinical nurse specialist. Surgical Nurse 6(3):21–25

Manley K (1997) A conceptual framework for advanced practice: an action research project operationalizing an advanced practitioner/nurse consultant role. Journal of Clinical Nursing 6(3):179–190

McGee P, Castledine G, Brown R (1996) A survey of specialist and advanced practice in England. Research report published by the Nursing Research Unit. University of Central England, Birmingham

McLoughlin S (1992) Congress on nursing practice meets. American Nurse 24:23

Ministry of Health and Scottish Home and Health Department (1966) Senior Nursing staff structure ('Salmon report') HMSO, London

NHS Executive (1999a) Making a difference: strengthening the nursing, midwifery and health visiting contribution to health and health care

NHS Executive (1999b) Nurse, midwife and health visitor consultants: establishing new posts and making appointments (appended with the UKCC higher level of practice pilot standards). Health Service Circular 217

NHS Executive (1999c) Nurse, midwife and health visitor consultants 1999/2000. Advanced Letter (NM) 2

NHS Executive (1998) Nurse consultants. Health Service Circular 161

NHS Executive (1999) Working together – securing a quality workforce for the NHS. Health Service Circular 79

NHS Management Executive (1992) Junior doctors: the new deal. NHSME, London

Royal College of Nursing (RCN) (1988) Specialties in nursing. RCN, London

School of Health and Related Research (SCHARR) (1999) Exploring new roles in practice: final report. SCHARR, University of Sheffield, Sheffield

Stilwell B (1985) Setting the scene: the nurse practitioner. Nursing Mirror 160(15):15–16

Touche Ross (1994) Evaluation of nurse practitioner projects in South Thames. NHS Executive/South Thames Regional Health Authority, London

United Kingdom Central Council for Nursing, Midwifery and Health Visiting (UKCC) (1992) The scope of professional practice. UKCC, London

United Kingdom Central Council for Nursing, Midwifery and Health Visiting (UKCC) (1994) The future of professional practice – the Council's standards for education and practice following registration. UKCC, London

Wilson-Barnett J (1995) Specialism in nursing: effectiveness and maximisation of benefit. Journal of Advanced Nursing 21(1) January:1–2

Woods L P (1998) Implementing advanced practice: identifying the factors that facilitate and inhibit the process. Journal of Clinical Nursing 7(3) May:265–273

An invisible revolution within the clinical team
New role development for the health-care professions

Ailsa Cameron   Lesley Doyal

Introduction

It may be tempting for those working in the 'new National Health Service (NHS)' to believe that it is only the nursing profession that has embarked on the road towards greater professional development and specialisation; but this is not the case. As the previous chapters have indicated, new role development is occurring within most health professions. This chapter draws on research evidence from the 'Exploring new roles in practice' project to illustrate the experiences of members of the health-care professions (HCPs) working in new roles. The chapter identifies some of the similarities between the experiences of HCPs and nurses as well as the differences that relate to the size and representation of these professions within acute care.

The policy context

The *Professions Supplementary to Medicine Act* was passed in 1960 in order to regulate the initial training and subsequent professional practice of a growing number of allied professions. The professions currently covered by the Act are: art, music and drama therapy; chiropody (podiatry); dietetics; medical laboratory science; occupational therapy; orthoptics; physiotherapy; prosthetics and orthotics; and radiography. The Council for the Professions Supplementary to Medicine was set up under the Act and through its professional boards now supervises the awarding of qualifications leading to state registration as well as monitoring the professional standards of individual practitioners. This legislation and its associated regulatory structure are currently under review and changes are expected soon.

Over the past few years there have been significant changes in the education and professional practice of the HCPs, with a gradual move towards higher education and graduate status for all new practitioners. All HCPs now have their own undergraduate education programmes, which are validated jointly by the higher education provider and the relevant professional body. As yet, in most institutions they do not share a common core of education but examples of multiprofessional educational programmes (such as the extensive shared learning pre-registration for occupational therapists and physiotherapists at the University of Southampton) are now beginning to emerge in individual institutions.

The total number of state registered HCPs is very small and even fewer currently work in the NHS. In 1998 there were approximately 105 327 state registered HCPs compared to 637 449 nurses. (This figure includes health visitors and midwives.) The relative size of these professions is important, particularly at a time when the composition of health services is being radically altered. In the context of the move from acute to primary care, for example, serious doubts are being raised about the future contribution of some professional groups. In 1996 a report from the University of Manchester

Health Services Management Unit on the future of the health-care workforce highlighted the pressure for change (Health Services Management Unit 1996). The 'Manchester report' argued for the creation of a generic health worker from which specialisms such as physiotherapy could emerge. Such debates can be interpreted as rather threatening to the smaller professions, whose education, role and skills are little understood by their professional colleagues, let alone the policy-making community.

Drivers for change – why are new roles being developed within the HCPs?

The emergence of new roles for the HCPs may be seen as a response to a variety of different drivers, not least the move towards greater autonomy and specialisation from within the professions.

However, the most powerful drivers for change (as in nursing) have come from external policy initiatives. These include:

◆ the impact of NHS reforms on the way in which services are configured
◆ the need to find more efficient and cost-effective means of providing services
◆ technological developments which allow therapists and nurses to carry out many procedures which in the past would have been undertaken by a doctor
◆ government initiatives such as moves to reduce waiting lists and the hours of work of junior doctors, which encouraged managers to think creatively about the composition of clinical teams and the allocation of work.

It is clear that factors of this kind will continue to have an impact on the practice of all professionals in the NHS. However, the challenges facing HCPs are in many senses unique because of their size, their low visibility and their lack of representation at senior levels within the decision-making processes.

Research evidence: the 'Exploring new roles in practice' project

In order to illustrate the implications of new role development within the HCPs this chapter draws on evidence from a number of case studies undertaken as part of the 'Exploring new roles in practice' project (ENRiP). The Department of Health, as part of its 'Human Resources Initiative', commissioned the ENRiP project in 1995. Its aim was to explore the extent of role development amongst nurses and HCPs working in acute care.

The ENRiP project had three stages. In Stage 1 a mapping exercise was conducted in a 20% sample of acute Trusts across England to identify the range and purpose of new role developments in nursing and the HCPs. For the purposes of the project 'new roles' were defined as those roles which had been identified by the participating Trusts as being innovative, non-traditional or taking on aspects of care previously performed by a different professional group, with the postholder having a nationally recognised qualification in a health profession. Information about these new roles was entered on a database, which was launched in 1997 (School of Health and Related Research 1997). In Stage 2 the database was used as the sampling frame for a set of case studies designed to explore the issues arising from the development of these new roles. In Stage 3 emergent themes were tested out on the total population of the database in order to establish their generalisability.

In this chapter the findings from the case studies undertaken by the University of Bristol are reported. These case studies were designed to explore new role development in the three largest HCP groups: physiotherapy, occupational therapy and radiography. Fourteen new roles were selected: three occupational therapists, seven physiotherapists, three diagnostic radiographers and one therapeutic radiographer. The posts were based in three acute hospitals: a teaching hospital (site J), an urban district general hospital (site L) and a rural district general hospital (site H). Details of the posts are given in Tables 6.1, 6.2 and 6.3.

Methodology

A case study approach was adopted, focusing on individual roles as the unit of investigation (Yin 1994). Through interviews with a range of different stakeholders it was possible to embed these individual case studies within a broader analysis of the NHS labour force in general and the HCPs in particular. This then enabled the wider issues related to the representation and management of HCPs in each of the Trusts to be explored.

Observational techniques were used as the initial means of collecting data about each of the individual roles. The aim of the observations was to allow the researchers to learn about the structure of the postholder's working day rather than to evaluate the clinical component of their work. Each postholder was then interviewed on a range of subjects that included personal biography, training, accountability, management support and future plans. Postholders were also asked to keep a reflective diary for 4 working weeks and to record any thoughts they had during that period that might be pertinent to a full understanding of their role.

Table 6.1 Characteristics of physiotherapy roles

Title and site	Grade	Post-registration qualifications	Recruitment process	Nature of employment	% time spent in role	Description
Respiratory physiotherapy specialist Site J	Super I	MSc	Post advertised externally, postholder interviewed	Full-time	100%	Postholder provides specialist advice, particularly on non-invasive ventilation. Research and education
Orthopaedic physiotherapy specialist Site J	Super I	MSc current	Covering post till externally advertised	Full-time	50%	Postholder sees patients referred to orthopaedic clinic for musculoskeletal assessment
Clinical physiotherapy specialist Site L	Super III Senior I (separate grades for each role)	–	Post advertised internally, postholder interviewed	Part-time	60%	Postholder has three roles: clinical physiotherapy specialist in pain education/management, orthopaedic specialist and outpatient physiotherapy
Physiotherapist – cardiac rehabilitation Site L	Super III	–	Postholder-developed post and service	Part-time	100%	Postholder manages cardiac rehabilitation service and provides specialist physiotherapy input to the service *(cont'd)*

Table 6.1 (cont'd)

Title and site	Grade	Post-registration qualifications	Recruitment process	Nature of employment	% time spent in role	Description
Senior physiotherapist – stroke discharge Site H	Senior I	–	Post advertised externally, postholder interviewed	Full-time	100%	Postholder provides specialist physiotherapy input to a multidisciplinary stroke discharge team
Senior physiotherapist rheumatology Site H	Senior I	–	Postholder asked by manager to work in role	Full-time	100%	Postholder provides specialist physiotherapy input to a multidisciplinary rheumatology team
Rheumatology clinical specialist Site H	Super II	MSc	Post advertised externally, postholder interviewed	Full-time	100%	Postholder provides specialist care for rheumatoid patients. Runs own clinics where she assesses and treats patients

Table 6.2 Characteristics of occupational therapy roles

Title and site	Grade	Post-registration qualifications	Recruitment process	Nature of employment	% time spent in role	Description
Occupational therapist – renal and orthopaedics Site J	Senior I	MSc	Post advertised externally, postholder interviewed	Full-time	50%	Postholder provides specialist advice and support to renal patients to ensure independence and safe discharge
Occupational therapist – cardiac rehabilitation Site L	Senior I		Postholder informally approached	Part-time	100%	Postholder provides occupational therapy input to the cardiac rehabilitation programme
Senior occupational therapist – stroke discharge Site H	Senior I		Post advertised externally, postholder interviewed	Full-time	100%	Postholder provides specialist occupational therapy input to a multidisciplinary stroke discharge team

Table 6.3 Characteristics of radiography (diagnostic and therapeutic) roles

Title and site	Grade	Post-registration qualifications	Recruitment process	Nature of employment	% time spent in role	Description
MRI radiographer Site J (diagnostic)	Super III	MSc current	Post advertised externally, postholder interviewed then promoted	Full-time	100%	Postholder responsible for day-to-day management of MRI unit. Trained to give IV injections
Clinic radiographer Site J (therapeutic)	Super IV	MDCR	Postholder asked by manager to work in role	Part-time	75%	Postholder coordinates care of breast cancer patients between units and clinic, also provides support and advice
MRI radiographer Site L (diagnostic)	Super III		Post advertised externally, postholder interviewed	Full-time	100%	Postholder responsible for day-to-day management of MRI unit. Trained to give IV injections
Radiographer Site H (diagnostic)	Basic grade		Postholder asked to train up	Full-time	100%	Postholder trained to give IV injections

Finally, interviews were conducted with heads of HCP services and the HCP executive representative at each site as a means of exploring issues about the individual posts and also to discuss the management, representation and future of the HCPs.

Basic findings

Models of practice

Postholders undertook a wide range of activities. Some tended towards the 'advanced practice' model of new role development in which clinical practice reaches beyond that of the mainstream profession to areas which may not be seen as the prerogative of the profession (Stewart 1998). Other posts were much more 'specialist' in their orientation (Chartered Society of Physiotherapy 1995). For example, posts like the orthopaedic physiotherapy specialist practitioner and the rheumatology clinical specialist were developed in order that a therapist rather than a doctor could assess patients in clinic and refer them on for further diagnostic tests or therapy treatment.

Most of the posts incorporated a diversity of activities in addition to clinical responsibilities. These often included supervisory, educational, research and management roles. Some also had responsibility for building up Trust business in their area of work from potential purchasers both inside and outside the NHS. For example, one of the magnetic resonance imaging (MRI) radiographers was developing a diagnostic service for a number of local private hospitals. Some of the managers spoke of actively developing roles that had a broad portfolio to ensure that these highly qualified professionals could contribute as much as possible to the work of their department.

Accountability

As in many new roles, patterns of accountability and line management were complex (Dowling et al 1996). Many of the postholders were not managed by members of their own profession. At site L the clinical physiotherapy specialist reported that she was managerially accountable to a psychologist when she worked in her role in pain education, the occupational therapist was responsible to the physiotherapist who ran the cardiac rehabilitation programme, while the cardiac rehabilitation physiotherapist herself was managerially accountable to the medical elderly services manager. The MRI radiographer, on the other hand, saw herself as managerially responsible to the radiologist running the particular session and to the business manager.

All but one of the 14 postholders studied regarded themselves as professionally accountable to their own profession's senior manager. However, clinical accountability was widely spread. The majority traced their clinical accountability to the consultant with whom they worked and only sometimes to a manager from their own profession.

To illustrate the complexity of these accountability arrangements let us consider again the practitioners working at site L, the urban district general hospital. The clinical physiotherapy specialist, who worked in three different roles, commented that she was clinically accountable to the physiotherapy manager when working in pain education, to the orthopaedic surgeon and physiotherapy manager when working in the orthopaedic outpatient clinic and to her physiotherapy manager when working in the outpatient clinic. The cardiac rehabilitation occupational therapist was clinically responsible to the cardiac rehabilitation physiotherapist, who herself was responsible to the consultant cardiologist. The MRI radiographer, on the other hand, saw herself as clinically responsible to the radiologist running the particular session and to the business manager who was a radiographer by background.

It appeared that practitioners had developed a complex matrix arrangement to deal with all aspects of their accountability. For those working in more than one role this could be a rather elaborate arrangement and was often the source of considerable concern.

Training and the assessment of competence

Previous research has identified the ad hoc nature of the training and preparation provided to nurses working in new roles (Doyal et al 1998). Not surprisingly we found a similar story for HCPs. When taking up their new roles, all the postholders had identified their educational needs and as a result the majority undertook some further training. However, the extent and aims of this training varied significantly. Most was in-house and tailored to the post itself rather than being generic and transferable. All the radiographers, for instance, were taught to give injections by either a doctor or nurse in their own Trust. Similarly those postholders, particularly physiotherapists who were working closely with medical colleagues in a role that might previously have been undertaken by a doctor, received some form of training from the consultant they worked with.

Assessment of competence in these new skills was also complex. Most of the assessments were undertaken by a doctor who would assess a particular skill rather than performance in the role overall. For example, the rheumatology clinical specialist received training from the consultant who led the team and was then assessed on her competence in completing specific procedures such as injecting joints rather than being assessed for all aspects of her role.

A number of the postholders commented that because they were breaking new ground for their profession no one knew what training they needed.

Some resolved this dilemma by contacting colleagues working elsewhere and putting together their own training packages. In general, education and training were complex and difficult areas with little clarity about what was required. In particular, problems arose from the lack of national awards or recognition, which undermined the confidence of these practitioners in their professional futures.

The experiences of individual postholders

Not surprisingly, these HCPs experienced many aspects of their new roles in ways similar to those reported by nurses in previous studies such as Doyal et al (1998). However, they also reported particular difficulties associated with their small numbers and with the general lack of knowledge amongst their clinical and managerial colleagues about HCPs and their education, training and preparation.

The challenge of a new role

Most regarded their new roles as an exciting challenge, commenting positively about what they hoped to achieve both for themselves and the wider profession. The respiratory physiotherapist said, 'I love it; it's not the label. I feel completely fulfilled from a professional point of view ... There should be more people like me, we have a lot to offer and can have a large input to patient management. It also enhances our reputation among other medical professions.'

Practitioners valued the greater autonomy the new posts had to offer whilst also recognising the increased pressures. At site L the cardiac rehabilitation physiotherapist summed up the contradictions very well: 'I am my own boss, I enjoy it, once you get the confidence in what you are doing ... I've said it myself, I like being my own boss and being on my own. On other occasions it's nice to get some support.'

Lack of clarity

Alongside this enthusiasm, however, there was a lack of clarity about the roles and what was expected of them. Postholders talked about their own confusion as well as that of colleagues and managers.

Indeed, when asked whether colleagues and other professionals understood their roles only 6 out of the 14 answered positively. This lack of comprehension about the new roles appeared to be compounded by the fact that the practitioners felt their colleagues did not understand the nature of their profession's contribution even in traditional settings. As the rheumatology physiotherapist at site H commented, 'I think consultants' understanding comes with time. General doctors don't know what physios and occupational therapists do. It took quite a long time for Dr X to understand what I could offer the service. Junior doctors, I think, pick up on what consultants refer but occasionally I get inappropriate referrals from juniors.'

Practitioners constantly talked about the need to educate others about their roles. The orthopaedic physiotherapy practitioner described how 'the consultants working alongside understand. The new registrars up there haven't worked with an orthopaedic physiotherapy practitioner so it's continually letting people know what you do ... I think they aren't aware of the experience and qualifications you've got to be there.' The stroke discharge physiotherapist working at site H described how the lack of understanding of her role could compromise clinical care: 'Nursing staff never know if I'm the ward physio or the stroke physio so I get the wrong referrals. I know some of the nursing staff are aware that I do things differently from other physios and they think it's because I'm new and don't know what to do. It's getting less as I am here longer.'

Postholders rarely mentioned any problems with communicating the nature of their role to patients. The clinical physiotherapy specialists remarked that 'It is easier [talking with patients] than talking to staff, mainly because they recognise the needs they have and the service you are offering meets their needs. They understand it and it's not really a problem.' Where there was a lack of comprehension this was linked to pre-existing confusion about the role of the HCPs themselves. However, the majority of postholders echoed the views of the rheumatology clinical specialist at site H who said, 'I don't think most of them [the patients] really know or care what you are so long as you are listening, caring and carrying out appropriate activities.'

Management support

For HCPs, as for nurses, concerns about identity and roles were often exacerbated by confusions about accountability and management support. The clinical physiotherapy specialist at site L said, 'I take patients from GPs now we are taking more responsibility. I feel supported but you do think something could explode. We have lost a bit of coat tail to hide under; it's new ground.' The cardiac rehabilitation physiotherapist on the same site described her situation as 'difficult, because nobody knows what I do or how I should do it, no one with specific experience who could help me as a professional [in] cardiac rehabilitation.'

Many of the postholders were managed by someone from another profession and this could lead to a number of difficulties, particularly with regard to the lack of professional support. The disappearance of professional teams meant that there was often no one to mentor individual postholders. At site H the stroke discharge physiotherapist felt that she had to go outside the hospital to get any kind of perspective on her clinical practice. 'I did 5 days' study leave and I organised myself to go to a rehabilitation centre in Surrey. The idea behind the training was to make sure my clinical practice was correct at the moment. I don't have a peer in the hospital with the same clinical area and experience so I am aware that nobody is able to be critical about my practice.'

The occupational therapist at site J said, 'I have got to the stage where I am a bit stuck. There is nobody other than X [the head occupational therapist] to discuss where I go to from here. I feel there should be other people to turn to … I know nursing has that facility.' The lack of management support often left these practitioners feeling isolated and 'adrift' from their professional colleagues.

Being unique

The problems of being unique were constantly stressed, particularly when discussing training issues. The clinical physiotherapy specialist said, 'There is no one else in a position to know what training we need', while the cardiac rehabilitation physiotherapist commented, 'It would have been nice to have more guidance but difficult for anyone to lead when it was evolving.' At site J the respiratory physiotherapist said, 'I feel I have little in common with the rest of the physios in my team and if my counterpart X wasn't here I'd have gone under – that's the one person I can have a moan to, we have different problems and the other offers support.'

Sometimes this lack of clarity led to a lack of acceptance of the practitioner by their professional colleagues. This was the case for the clinic radiographer, who commented that 'because it was a new role and was something they hadn't experienced some people find it hard to accept that a radiographer can do something different than they would traditionally do. I wouldn't say the whole department is behind it as a necessary task … Some call me a skin nurse to wind me up.' Working in a new role could be a lonely and difficult experience.

In discussing their experiences, the postholders often referred to wider professional debates illustrating significant differences between nurses and HCPs. In nursing, debates about new roles have dominated the mainstream professional literature and the activities of the statutory and professional organisations for many years. In the HCPs, however, the debate about changing forms of practice appears to be less well developed and this had an impact on individual practitioners, making it more difficult for them to get clear and consistent advice on issues such as titles and grading.

The respiratory physiotherapist at site J sought clarity from the Chartered Society of Physiotherapy (CSP) about the grading of specialist posts and the guidance being sent out. However, she received little help. 'What is the difference between a clinical specialist and physiotherapy practitioner? The CSP didn't know.' Later she reported some progress: 'Good news on the "clinical specialist" and "practitioner" problem. My boss sees me as a clinical practitioner with day-to-day routine case-load responsibilities ... at last some direction! I will photocopy the guidelines and bring them up at our own specialist meetings.'

Future careers

Many of the HCPs in this study were concerned about their future careers. The nature of their posts and the ad hoc status of their training put question marks over any future moves. Most were clear about what they saw as the benefits of having worked in an innovative role. Working in a new role had made them 'different' and therefore probably attractive to future employers. As one of the MRI radiographers said, 'I think it is a good post to have come from, it will make me a favourable candidate because I built the post and service from scratch so I think it will set me up favourably.' The orthopaedic physiotherapy practitioner took a similar view, saying, 'It's a good post to do even for 3 or 4 months because they are not common posts so having it on the CV is a good thing.'

The rheumatology physiotherapist said, 'I'm glad I'm in a specialty because it has forced me into developing and I think by developing I will secure my professional future. My gut feeling is if you are a jack of all trades when they employ less physios the writing is on the wall for them but I may be doing an [ostrich] of burying my head. Can't tell what is round the corner.' However, the clinic radiographer felt that stepping outside her normal area of practice might have compromised her chances of future employment. She said, 'I think being outside of mainstream radiography doesn't do you much good. It's great for a short time but if I stayed out of mainstream clinical radiotherapy I think it would be hard to maintain your grading if I were to go to a post elsewhere that was clinical.'

The reality was that all were in relatively innovative posts in changing professions and no one could be sure about the future. The qualifications and experience they were gaining were not part of a recognised career structure and this could be a source of considerable anxiety.

The management and representation of HCPs within acute Trusts

Management arrangements

The arrangements for managing individual new posts and HCP services varied between Trusts. There was no single model but two characteristics were consistent across all sites. All radiographers were managed independently of the other HCPs in separate units and all occupational therapists were represented at senior management level, either formally or informally, by a physiotherapist.

At site J, the teaching hospital, physiotherapists and occupational therapists were based in a therapies directorate and were represented at Trust board level by the clinical services director (a doctor). Radiographers were based in diagnostic imaging and were also represented at the Trust board by the clinical services director. Therapeutic radiographers were based in oncology and represented at executive level by the clinical director of cancer services.

In discussing the effectiveness of these arrangements a number of the respondents emphasised the problem of the relatively small size of their professional group. They also compared the power of HCPs with that of nurses. One therapy manager was particularly bothered that the clinical director was a doctor. 'Doctors don't understand other roles. Therefore they have no concepts to understand HCPs with ... Nursing has accessed the system much better, so there is no room for the rest of us so we are never at the top of her agenda. It doesn't work.'

Similarly, the occupational therapy manager at the same site claimed that her role was made difficult by the failure to understand the role of occupational therapists. 'We are constantly having to teach new people about each other's roles. Occupational therapy is much better recognised in mental health; we are constantly having to redefine our role and market ourselves.' The radiography manager said, 'Being in clinical services is mostly good but people do forget about us because we are not at the acute interface. We're seen as a service industry. They ask us to do things and expect us to do it; it's a fault across the Trust.'

The clinical services director herself felt that HCPs were not adequately represented in the Trust. She was concerned about inequities between staff groups in their access to development funds and also felt concerned that they did not have easy access to her. She admitted that 'they get forgotten. Nurses and doctors have their specific representatives but PAMs don't. I hadn't really thought of myself as the PAMs' executive representative until you mentioned it.'

At the remaining two sites management arrangements were similarly complex, but at both sites the nurse executive represented physiotherapists and occupational therapists at board level. However, one of the nurse executives herself remarked that HCPs were not adequately represented. She described how 'At the moment they are not represented at all ... They have special needs and it is easy to see them outside the mainstream of patient care. In future they will be represented separately. I will talk about them on the Board and raise their profile. They will have access to the Trust things we've done for nurses in terms of education. Maybe that's why the therapies grumble because they don't have profile but they are so important.' She saw occupational therapists as especially vulnerable: 'You can see how they are sitting because they are represented by a physio; you don't hear occupational therapists talking about themselves in the Trust, but [we] can't do without them especially in rehabilitation. When services are off-site they are out of mind ... You have to increase their profile and show how valuable they are.'

New roles and existing career structures

Alongside their discussions of the overall arrangements the various managers were also asked about the implications of HCP career structures for the development of new roles. Not surprisingly, the managers picked up on a number of concerns mentioned by the postholders themselves. They were aware that the existing career structures were not appropriate for the new roles and needed further attention from employers and professional bodies. At site J the head of therapies spoke particularly of new roles for physiotherapists, saying, 'It is difficult to get a grading structure to reward them appropriately. We want a grading structure that will work across all the PAMs. They are expensive people.' The radiotherapy manager also talked about pay and about the problems of accrediting new roles. 'Doctors get paid more so shouldn't this be rewarded better? Yes, accreditation and certification of extended roles ... Doctors don't want academic courses because they want to supervise the extended role themselves.'

When asked about the future career prospects of their new postholders managers were not always positive. Radiography and physiotherapy managers in particular talked about the problems of practitioners becoming too narrowly focused. The head of radiotherapy at site J was positive but also sounded some warnings: 'If someone came to me with those skills I'd really like to employ them. However, it would have to be another place [Trust] that needs those type of skills.' The head of radiography at the same site was the most negative but also seemed to have the broadest view of the career implications for postholders. Speaking of the radiographer working in MRI, she said, 'It depends on how long she stays in it. I think she needs to broaden her horizons ... She's been doing MRI for a while now ... The logical step would be to go to a bigger MRI department; she's developed some management skills. In the main department she could have more global responsibilities but she hasn't latched on to it yet ... She only manages three or four people and would have to drop down grades if she went into general radiography work.'

At site H physiotherapists were picked out for particular comment by the head of therapies. 'I think it can only enhance career development but unfortunately if you are a clinical specialist you get to Senior 1 and there is nowhere else to go on clinical grading. It is fairly rigid here.' At site L all four of the therapy managers thought the posts they supervised needed broadening if the postholders were to benefit fully. The head of physiotherapy commented that 'they could do something similar elsewhere but it is probably limiting rather than expanding as they are very narrow fields. They could become experts in wider fields.'

The radiography manager at site L also identified remuneration issues. 'It is difficult. Specialist superintendents are in a difficult situation; if they want to stay in clinical areas these roles are a dead end. We need to recognise that and broaden her role and keep her motivated, keep her professionally up to date. In terms of reward it's a dead end. I'd like to see a technical pay scale alongside management pay scale. There is no financial benefit. It's sad; there should be mechanisms to reward that.'

The future

The challenges facing HCPs in the new NHS are in many senses unique because of their numbers, their low visibility and their lack of representation. Although they are subject to many of the same forces for change that other professional groups face they also have their own particular characteristics both as a group of small professions occupying a specific position within the structure of the NHS and as individual professions within this larger grouping. These characteristics will have a significant effect on how they are able to respond to current challenges both generally and with respect to the development of new roles.

One of the most significant professional developments within the NHS has been the move towards evidence-based practice. Though there will continue to be debate about both its technical and its value base, evidence-based practice will continue to be regarded as the only acceptable mode of operation in health care. Ensuring evidence-based practice will mean that all professions will need to justify not just particular interventions and ways of working but also quite possibly their own continued existence as a distinct group of workers. Part of this process of justification will require greater attention to be paid by all health professionals to the cluster of activities relating to audit, research and effectiveness. This trend may be of particular importance to the sustainability of the new professional roles which cross professional boundaries. Whether these posts are at the therapist/medicine interface or the nursing/therapist interface they will come under increasing pressure to demonstrate their clinical and cost-effectiveness.

Occupational therapy

From these research findings, the professional group that appears to be most at risk from future developments is occupational therapy. The changing nature of health care has led to radical changes both in the patterns of care delivered by occupational therapists, and in their place of work. As hospital stays have declined and care in the community has increased, occupational therapists have experienced a shift away from 'hands-on' rehabilitation work towards assessment, evaluation and discharge planning.

The significance of these developments for the profession has been profound and has marked a fundamental change in the nature of occupational therapists' clinical practice (Cameron & Masterson 1998). Occupational therapists in particular have been caught in a trap where they need to justify their continuation as an independent profession while at the same time responding as flexibly as possible to the changes going on around them. This has led to a situation where their distinctive contribution has often been obscured and their new work increasingly overlaps with that of other professional groups.

This situation appears to be exacerbated by the fact that many occupational therapists are now managed by physiotherapists, who generally seem to have achieved greater status within the new NHS Trusts. Of all the HCP groups, occupational therapy also seems to be furthest from the medical power base. This has further weakened their capacity to market their services and determine their own practice.

Physiotherapy

Physiotherapists face similar problems. This is particularly evident in those areas where new roles have been created that could be occupied by either nurses or physiotherapists. In respiratory medicine and rheumatology, aspects of the therapeutic role are being reconfigured in ways that do not conform to the traditional occupational boundaries between physiotherapists, specialist nurses and doctors. As a result the distinctive contribution of particular professions will come under increasing scrutiny and this is likely to be reinforced by the growing emphasis on audit and evidence-based practice. Thus physiotherapists face many of the same challenges as their colleagues in occupational therapy. However, they are probably in a stronger position since they are more likely to be in senior management positions and they appear to have maintained a closer relationship with the medical profession.

Radiography

The situation of the radiography profession seems to be different. Radiography tends to have closer links to medicine and has also managed to maintain its own line management structure. Most radiographers are managed from within their own profession with representation to the board usually being through a doctor. The work of radiographers is more clearly understood by most doctors and they are seen to have 'harder' and more 'scientific' knowledge than the other HCPs.

Diagnostic radiographers have expanded into new roles with greater autonomy. They work independently both in primary care settings and in accident and emergency, and are also being given significant responsibilities in the operation of new technologies such as MRI, computed tomography and ultrasound. However, these developments have highlighted the boundary problem between the work of radiologists and radiographers. While there has been little concern from medical colleagues about radiographers carrying out procedures such as barium enemas, their increasing role in reporting on images has been viewed with suspicion. The significant overlap between the skills of radiographers and radiologists and the potential for radiographers to take over more high-status tasks raise a number of questions about future relations between the two professions.

At the same time, nurses are acquiring some of the skills traditionally seen to belong to radiographers. In the area of ultrasonography, many nurses and midwives are coming to regard the use of this technology as a routine part of their jobs, raising issues about the boundaries between radiography and nursing. Thus as diagnostic radiographers try to extend their roles they are to some extent being 'squeezed' between radiologists above them and nurses coming alongside. These boundary disputes will need resolution. However, diagnostic radiographers as a group are unlikely to face any significant challenge to their position, as diagnostic imaging becomes increasingly central to the practice of acute care.

In the case of therapeutic radiography, however, things look much less certain. The changing nature of oncology practice has posed serious challenges to this very small professional group. In particular the recommendations of the Expert Advisory Group on Cancer will require significant changes in how and where services are provided. For many therapeutic radiographers the main development of their role has been towards a more 'holistic' approach, with counselling becoming a major part of their activities. However, this moves them away from their technical training and 'scientific' knowledge base to one already colonised by nurses. Thus there is again a blurring of boundaries and a lack of clarity about the implications of new roles for the longer-term professional future of therapeutic radiography.

Conclusion

This chapter has demonstrated some of the similarities and differences in relation to new role development between the occupational therapy, physiotherapy and radiography professions. All of these professions are facing the challenges of a changing NHS from a very small professional base. The roles discussed in this chapter have played an important part in demonstrating the potential contribution of health-care professionals to new patterns of health care. At the same time, however, they raise important questions about current professional boundaries, about specialisation and genericism and about the future not just of traditional HCP career structures but even of the professions themselves.

REFERENCES

Cameron A, Masterson A (1998) The changing policy context of occupational therapy. British Journal of Occupational Therapy 61(12):556–560

Chartered Society of Physiotherapy (CSP) (1995) Specialisms and specialists. Information paper no PA23. CSP, London

Dowling S, Martin R, Skidmore P et al (1996) Nurses taking on junior doctors' work: a confusion of accountability. British Medical Journal 312:1211–1214

Doyal L, Dowling S, Cameron A (1998) Challenging practice: an evaluation of four innovatory nursing posts in the South West. Policy, Bristol

Health Services Management Unit (1996) The future healthcare workforce. University of Manchester, Manchester

School of Health and Related Research (SCHARR) (1997) The ENRiP data base. SCHARR, University of Sheffield, Sheffield

Stewart M (1998) Advanced practice in physiotherapy. Physiotherapy 84(4):184–186

Yin R K (1994) Case study research. Sage, London

7

The consumer perspective

Tina Funnell

Introduction

'If patients don't change health care, who will?' This simple yet powerful question was a recurring theme at the Patient's Charter Conference held in 1995 in Georgia, USA. Modern health-care systems can be bewilderingly complex and in trying to balance the dimensions of cost, quality and access to ensure optimum outcomes, the patients' interests and needs have too often been obscured. Patients are first and foremost human beings with human hopes and needs, not simply diseases with a person attached. Increasingly patients want to take a more active role in determining the nature of their health care. They want to work as partners with health professionals rather than being passive recipients of services. In the foreword to 'A first-class service' (Department of Health 1998) the Secretary of State for Health emphasises the need for a health service that is delivered with courtesy and which has a real understanding of patient's fears and worries.

The points raised in this chapter draw heavily on my own experiences spanning over 20 years as a consumer representative in health care. Some consumer representatives have taken the view that the patient's perspective is the only one that matters and in so doing have devalued the clinical expertise of the health professions. In the end the patients' expectations and values have to be the overriding guide to the decisions that are made about treatment and the benefits and side-effects of those treatments. Yet it would be far better if these decisions were made jointly by everyone involved so that patients and the health professionals contribute their knowledge and understanding as equals. Patients and their carers would then have the best and most impartial information available to make choices and decisions that really are relevant to them and their lifestyle.

About me

First let me tell you a little about where I am coming from and in particular one area of work with which I am involved so that you can set my comments into some sort of context. I was actively involved in one patient organisation – the National Eczema Society – for 20 years until I moved on from being chief executive in December 1996. I started as a member because my youngest child had severe eczema, then I became involved as a holiday organiser and finally I was chief executive for 16 years. During this time I always worked closely with clinical colleagues, recognising that partnerships were vital if patients and their carers are to have available to them impartial, accurate, evidence-based and comprehensive information to manage and live with a chronic long-term condition, as best as they could.

The UK has a long tradition of voluntary organisations and charities working together. It was not surprising therefore that, when the 1990 *NHS and Community Care Act* reforms (Department of Health 1990) began to be implemented four patient organisations worked together to form an umbrella organisation for patients with chronic, long-term, fluctuating incurable disorders: the Long-term Medical Conditions Alliance. As one of the founder members I was active in the early years and served as chair of this group for 2 years. The organisation now has 100 patient groups in membership. In addition, I have acted amongst other things as a patient adviser to the All-Party Parliamentary Group on Skin. I was also a member of the Standing Advisory Group on Consumer Involvement in the NHS Research and Development Programme and a member of the NHS Patient Partnership Working Group. I am now chair of the Consumer Health Information Centre and organising secretary of the Health Coalition Initiative.

Most of what I will say in this chapter is based therefore on my extensive experience of working with people with chronic, long-term, fluctuating, incurable conditions. This group of patients is where most of the work of patient support groups and disease-focused patient groups is concentrated. Despite having many different diseases, however, patients have many common problems to face. The traditional medical model with its focus on cure often has little to offer these patients, who have to live with their condition for life, and often all aspects of their lives are affected. They are often vulnerable to other, sometimes contradictory, sources of information and advice such as health pages in magazines and newspapers, complementary and alternative therapists, the Internet and family and friends. Many of the larger patient groups raise funds for research and also employ clinical specialists such as nurses and members of the health-care professions (HCPs).

The patient

No discussion of the consumer perspective would be complete without an analysis of the patient within this perspective. What is the patient exactly? In my opinion the patient is not merely a clinically interesting blob that comes into the hospital, sits in a bed, has things done to it and then walks out well again. Equally patients are not their disease – not a cancerous tumour or an irritable bowel, for example; nor are they victims, people to be pitied, guinea pigs, problems or burdens. Yet much of the language and methods health professionals have traditionally used when dealing with patients demonstrates that this is exactly how they have been seen. Patients are human beings with a range of responsibilities and roles in life, who happen to have a part of the body or mind that is not functioning well and which prevents them from leading normal lives the way they want to. In other words patients are not a homogeneous group with a clear identity and set views, or the same standards and expectations of care and treatment. Patients are people just like you and me but unfortunately they are often still viewed in terms of the old health-care model – that is, as objects of care rather than active participants in that care.

I find it useful to think of patients in four broad groups, each of which indicates a different set of health-care needs and demands a different relationship with the health professions. First there is the person who has a one-off episode like a heart attack. If I had a heart attack now, I would not wish to have a debate with the health professionals about how they were going to treat me and what my options were. I would make the assumption that they know exactly what to do, that they are up to date with new developments and that they have accurate knowledge about the benefits and risks of the various treatments available to me. However, when I am recovered enough to go home, I need support, information, advice and a realistic prognosis to enable me to continue to lead a full, active and healthy life.

The second group consists of people with chronic long-term conditions. Managing people with long-term, fluctuating, incurable conditions such as eczema, asthma, manic depression and diabetes presents the health services with a major challenge. These people live with their diseases their whole lives, and as a result will have long-term relationships with their health professionals and health services. In addition, because such patients live with their conditions over a long period of time, they frequently know more about the condition and its impact on their lives than the staff who care for them. This can be quite threatening for professionals, who are often considered or who consider themselves 'the experts'. However, it can also be used positively and beneficially if the professionals are sensitive to the importance that people with long-term conditions attach to their relationships with professionals. These life-long patients – and many of you are working with them – are dependent on medications and treatments for their ability to lead as normal a life as possible, so they attach great importance to the efficacy of these treatments. If health professionals involve such patients in understanding their treatment and the benefits that they can realistically expect, and emphasise the fact that they are not cures but techniques of management, this will increase self-management and confidence. People with chronic long-term conditions will bear huge 'other' costs which are often not considered by health professionals. Such patients bear significant financial, social and psychological costs because their diseases have an impact on all aspects of life – on the patients' lives as well as those of their family, peers and work colleagues, if they are lucky enough to be in work. For example, the financial consequences of a long-term disease such as eczema are huge. In addition to the cost of medications and treatments, there are the added costs of buying extra clothing and bedding because of the staining caused by blood and creams, the extra household chores to keep allergens at bay and the replacement costs of washing machines and dryers which wear out more quickly. There is also the loss of time from work for hospital appointments.

The third group consists of those patients with one-off 'minor' complaints who often present to the doctor or nurse practitioner in the health centre or accident and emergency department. They are sometimes described as the 'worried well', 'inappropriate attenders' or 'trivia' – what a put-down these terms are! They are nevertheless people who have decided that they need support, advice or intervention from a health professional. Health professionals must recognise that even though such patients' measures and values may be different from those of the clinicians they are still of equal importance. The Consumer Health Information Centre aims to help the public increase its understanding of common ailments and how they can be self-managed.

Approximately 60% of visits to GPs are for minor ailments. Compared with research carried out in the 1980s consumers in the late 1990s increasingly report that they are willing and interested in managing their own ill health. However, one of the biggest barriers to self-treatment is a lack of knowledge, particularly in relation to 'diagnosing' the problem. An increasing number of medications, which were formerly only available on prescription, are now available over the counter in chemists. This trend is likely to continue and so it will be increasingly important for consumers to be equipped to make an informed decision about the products they purchase and to see the pharmacist as a key health professional from whom they may seek such advice.

The fourth group is composed of those patients with terminal illnesses. For these patients, care of the family is essential. Their ability and confidence to continue their lives after the death of the family member will be greatly affected by the sensitivity and support they are offered during their contact with the health service.

Challenging traditional conceptions of care

Twenty to thirty years ago many patients with conditions such as muscular dystrophy and cystic fibrosis would not have survived. Drug therapy and improved therapeutic interventions have prolonged life. Similarly, the prevalence of diseases such as asthma and eczema has increased exponentially, which has tremendous resource implications for the health service. Despite policy exhortations to the contrary, the health service still runs on a very medical model founded on notions of cure and treatment. The doctor, despite the claims of the nursing and HCPs' professional organisations, is still seen as the leader and services are structured around disease conditions, systems of the body and types of medical intervention. Patients and their carers, however, want and need holistic approaches. For example, many patients with eczema also have asthma and often are dealt with by two completely separate health-care teams, necessitating two sets of clinic appointments, whereas the development of an asthma/eczema specialist team would be far more appropriate.

While many patients still prefer to leave all decisions to the health professionals and do not feel able to question medical advice, growing numbers are not content simply to hand over responsibility for their health, as the following quotation from a member of the Swedish Cystic Fibrosis Association demonstrates:

> We need to clearly identify who the professional is and when is the doctor the professional and when am I, the patient, the professional because I have the disease? Most cystic fibrosis patients, for example, receive care

from a specialist, and there may be only one in the country. If the patient with cystic fibrosis then gets another illness, say measles, he or she visits the family doctor. The doctor may not know how to treat a cystic fibrosis patient who has measles because he or she does not know what antibiotic treatment this type of patient should have. In this case the patient goes to the doctor and pays but actually tells him what to do. That is the way we function very often. So the question has to be: 'who is the professional and when?'. Doctors are professionals but so are patients.

Patients, particularly those with long-term health conditions, have often become expert about their bodies and their disease and understandably feel hurt and resentful if this expertise is not respected and used positively to manage their conditions. This expertise can, however, be very threatening to traditional health professionals who see themselves as the experts. In addition the patients' needs for information and support in relation to living a full and active life may not be considered to be important because they fall outside of the strictly medical definitions of need. Nurses and HCPs therefore can provide an important link between medicine and what the patient/client/carer actually needs and wants. Nurses and HCPs, particularly those working in new clinical roles, need to work with patients to reshape our health services and encourage patients to be equal partners in their health care, with as much or as little responsibility as they can handle.

Rethinking services

Despite commitments from both the professions and policy-makers, services still tend to be organised for the benefit of the professionals rather than the patient. For example, the mention of open access clinics usually brings the stock answer that hospitals and health centres will be flooded with people with minor problems demanding treatment there and then. However, evidence from consumer organisations demonstrates the opposite. For example, I vividly remember a member of the Eczema Society describing the dramatic change in her and her son's life since moving home. At her first place of residence her son had monthly appointments with the consultant; this involved her taking a day off work and her son missing a day from school, often to wait for a considerable time, to have a few minutes' consultation whether they needed it or not. On moving they went to see the new dermatologist who, after a detailed assessment, told them to ring when they needed treatment and they would be slotted into the weekly eczema clinic. A year later they had visited only once when the son's eczema had rapidly become infected after a sudden flare. Mum recognised the problem and he was seen promptly. The son had treatment when he needed it, whereas with the first hospital they would have had to wait for the regular appointment or see the GP. The family felt happier because they were in control of their own lives, the mother was not losing money and/or holiday time from having to take unnecessary time off work and the son was able to concentrate on his exams. In addition, rather than increasing demand, the hospital had been able to offer 11 consultations to other people who needed them. Different doesn't always imply more.

Education

One important way in which patient groups can contribute to the skills and knowledge of health-care professionals is by participating in their education. We need to ensure that education for health professionals is focused on patient need rather than professional perceptions of need. Why, for instance, is there such a woeful lack of investment in research and development, training and education for some of the long-term chronic conditions such as skin disease? After all, 20% of the population will have a skin problem at some time in their lives and it is estimated that approximately 10% of general practice consultations are concerned with skin problems. Yet dermatology is not a core subject in medical or nursing schools and there are only 319 dermatologists in the UK. Many nurses and doctors can complete their professional education without knowing anything about dermatology. To try to address this gap the National Eczema Society has developed patient-centred educational programmes for health professionals, with some unanticipated positive effects as demonstrated by the following quotation from a nurse who attended one of these courses:

> The most important aspect was that, as a parent of a child with eczema, I have been told about eczema and shown some of the treatments available. In 9 years of dealing with my daughter's eczema we have never once been shown how to use cream or lotions and never been told the importance of re-hydrating the skin and keeping it moisturised. Since this study day I have felt confident in the way I treat my daughter's eczema, and it certainly shows because since then we have had *no* flare ups.

Advocacy and empowerment

Debates continue to reverberate in the policy and professional literature about what to call patients. People with health needs have been called 'patients', 'clients', 'users and carers', 'consumers' and now, as they increasingly pay for services, 'customers'. You cannot change a patient into a consumer just by changing the name, however; the power balance too must be altered. Also, evidence from patients' organisations suggests that 'patient' is the correct word because it is what people prefer to be called. Being a consumer or even a customer implies you have a choice. The essence of consumerism is that consumers should get what they want, not what producers choose to offer. We have choice when we shop in a store because we can make our own judgements about what we want. In most industries the consumer makes the purchasing decisions and pays for the products or services. In health care, the purchasing decision, payment and receipt of services are separated. Well-functioning competition is characterised by demanding consumers with enough clout to push providers to improve quality, while at the same time reducing costs, but when customers are fragmented, as they are in health care, their power is greatly diminished. Health-care consumers also lack access to the information that would improve their decisions and in turn enable them to pressurise providers to improve care while reducing costs. In most industries customers can compare product performance and price. Health care is very different. Patients and health professionals do not readily have access to meaningful measures of quality for interventions and treatment options. However, the introduction of the National Institute for Clinical Excellence and the developing framework that clinical governance provides will hopefully begin to address this.

Nurses and HCPs tend to see their role as that of an advocate *for* patients. Instead they should be standing alongside patients to enable them to negotiate for the most appropriate services and care. To do this there needs to be respect for each other's knowledge. Health professionals, for example, often have a little knowledge about many individual situations whereas the patient has a lot of knowledge about a single situation. That does not invalidate either set of knowledge – each has its value and must be respected. That patients should be treated as partners in the health-care process is a concept that is now being enshrined in various documents including the World Health Organization's 'Declaration of the promotion of patients' rights in Europe' which was agreed in Amsterdam in 1994 (WHO 1994).

Much research has been carried out on relationships between health professionals and patients but almost exclusively this has been done from the health professionals' perspective. We need further work on the patient part of this relationship. An understanding of what patients expect to receive from the health-care process is needed. The system has to be sensitive to the fact that patient expectations will not be met if patients cannot effectively tell health-care professionals what they want. For example, in eczema management, a mother with severe hand eczema may be far more concerned that she is not managing her baby well than she is about her eczema. Perhaps she cannot bathe the baby because her hands are too sore. If she does not receive help with that very practical matter, she will go home from her consultation with the health professional very distressed although she may have received good help with the pure clinical aspect of managing eczema. As this example demonstrates, patients rarely need or want to challenge the clinical competence of health professionals but do wish to broaden their focus beyond the purely clinical element of the disease. It may well be that the survey of NHS users being undertaken by the Department of Health will begin to provide a wider perspective for the service of what consumers are really seeking from it.

Patient associations

Most patient associations and consumer groups are membership organisations. Sometimes several work in the same disease area. Each will have its particular emphasis, culture, policy, issues and aims and there may even be rivalries between groups. Although some devote considerable funds to research into their particular disease, arguably their most important contribution is their accumulated knowledge of how patients perceive their condition and its management. They must also develop skills to ensure that they truly reflect the views of a wide range of patients and carers and such consultations involve time, effort and patience. Patient associations and consumer groups fall into three major types in terms of size and income. There are large bodies such as the British Diabetic Association and the Multiple Sclerosis Society with substantial income and perhaps a professional team, able to take advantage of marketing, public relations and fundraising. Then there are medium-sized organisations such as the Eczema Society dealing with diseases that do not attract huge resources but which have to cope with the demands placed on them. Finally there are many small groups such as the Psoriatic Arthropathy Alliance or Bechet's Syndrome which depend heavily on volunteer staff.

With some exceptions groups that represent patients are most often disease-specific and their activities emphasise the specific needs of patients with that disease. Comprehensive and appropriate service development, however, requires the development of alliances that transcend specific concerns and focus on system-wide improvements in health care.

As the voluntary and charitable sector expands there are recurring debates about its future. In this changing and challenging environment how do patient organisations balance ideals, imperatives, aims and needs? How do they balance working on behalf of patients and consumers with being major providers of services? If much of their income comes from fees for providing services how do they balance the need to maintain that income with speaking out, which might jeopardise their funding? If advocacy groups do not empower patients and consumers, who will? Few organisations have the means to respond to every request for patients to be involved in consultations where a patient view is now required. As the NHS through its patient partnership initiatives has promoted the need for patients and carers to be more involved in decision-making at every level, so pressure has increased on organisations to find representatives, not only nationally but locally and regionally, which is time-consuming and expensive and which the NHS often treats as free goods. Finding appropriate representation can also be difficult. If representation is tokenistic or inappropriate little real benefit will be gained and all the participants may find the process a frustrating and negative experience. The umbrella organisations such as the Long-Term Medical Conditions Alliance (LMCA), Genetic Interest Group, Neurological Alliance and the Primary Immunodeficiency Association can often play a useful role in advocating and representing patient views.

New role development

Nurses and HCPs are increasingly reshaping their practice and sharing a skills base with other colleagues in health and social care. Practitioners, together with colleagues, are determining the most appropriate models of local service delivery and as a consequence professional boundaries are becoming less distinct and new clinical roles are being developed. Patients must become more involved in setting standards for assessing the quality of care and the professionals who provide it.

It is in this context that I was delighted to join the United Kingdom Central Council for Nursing, Midwifery and Health Visiting (UKCC) Steering Group looking at the regulation of 'A higher level of practice in nursing, midwifery and health visiting'. The UKCC's purpose is to establish and improve standards of nursing, midwifery and health visiting in order to serve and protect the public. The proposals are intended to safeguard the interests of the public and to meet their needs for competent practitioners who are working in these new ways and at higher levels than previously. Such development is urgently needed as the nature of work undertaken by all health-care professionals continues to change in response to the needs of users and developments in research, technology and practice.

Such measures of quality and those who assess it must be separate and independent from those who provide care. Full involvement by patients requires information that is readily accessible through a variety of media, comprehensive, easily understandable and relevant to the individual patient or carer. Creating and providing information, particularly about standards and treatment options, should be an interactive process between patients and health-care professionals.

A growing range of patient groups now fund new role developments, many of which are in nursing, e.g. Parkinson's disease nurses, the Multiple Sclerosis (MS) Society nurse specialists and the now well-established Macmillan Cancer

Relief nurses. In the case of Macmillan Cancer Relief, whilst the charity provides only pump-priming funding, these roles have become so central to the delivery of cancer care that it would be difficult to continue to run services without the support of this sector. The NHS has become extremely dependent on these 'pots of money' from charities to deliver core services. Yet the evidence base on which these organisations invest their funding resource, which is often raised by donation, is extremely limited at present and often shaped by a professional view of what is needed. This does, however, appear to be changing. In 1999 the MS Society developed a programme of partnership funding to support NHS Trusts seeking to establish MS nurse specialist posts. The society also provided an education package for professionals and published a national clinical guideline on the care and management of people with MS. Alongside this investment in service provision, the Society commissioned a 2-year external evaluation of the posts to inform future funding decisions.

Funds to support these types of development come mainly from donations, flag days, local fundraisers and volunteers. Whether these financial resources are being deployed to greatest benefit for patients is unclear. In the future not only will this question need to be more explicitly addressed through research but patient organisations may also decide that their funds could be more appropriately used in other ways. If, as the research seems to suggest, information is one of the keys to self-care then patient groups in the future may choose to invest in information experts and services. They may get involved in kite-marking World Wide Web resources and begin to realise the potential that digital technology offers for providing interactive patient-led services via the TV in people's homes.

From paternalism to partnership

I have been actively involved in work with Pharmaceutical Partners UK. This involved organising a series of workshops and seminars to promote partnerships and understanding between voluntary health organisations and the pharmaceutical industry. As a result of this work we produced a booklet entitled 'Making partnerships work'. The foreword was written by Baroness Pitkeathley (who was then chief executive of the Carers' National Association) and Edward Roberts (who was then chair of Pharmaceutical Partnerships for Better Healthcare). This guidance document identified some key principles of partnership. Although it is intended to promote best practice between the pharmaceutical industry and voluntary health organisations, the principles identified have a resonance with the types of relationship that nurses and HCPs taking on new roles should endeavour to engender with consumers of their services. The three principles that lie at the heart of productive partnerships are equity, transparency and mutual benefit.

Equity indicates that each of the partners is given due respect and recognition of his or her skills and values. Regular appraisal of aims and open acknowledgement of each partner's contribution must be seen as adding value to developing new roles and services. Transparency concerns the need to develop an atmosphere of openness and honesty. This may take time to build but is vital to ensure that patients' and carers' needs are met. Mutual benefit is an acknowledgement that partnerships are only sustainable if everyone involved sees the benefit to him or herself. Partners must understand and commit themselves to meeting each other's requirements as well as their own.

Traditionally health-care professionals have made all the decisions and patients have passively accepted these without question, but this is changing. While many patients still prefer to leave all decisions to the health-care professionals and do not feel able to question their advice, growing numbers are not content simply to hand over responsibility for their health. Also, as the focus of health-care practice shifts from illness to wellness health professionals will increasingly be working with active well-informed patients and carers who live with and manage their own health problems. One of the major challenges for new role development is ensuring that health-care professionals' knowledge of disease and its treatment and patients' knowledge and understanding about themselves and their conditions are brought together.

Conclusion

My vision is for a health service that is truly patient-centred, where patients make an equal contribution to health-care decisions, and where patients' views and needs are acted on, valued, respected and understood. To achieve this vision we must ensure appropriate patient representation at the various decision-making levels and processes within our health services and to accomplish this we must change the health-care culture to provide a more equitable distribution of power. There is already much to feel good about, such as the generally positive relationships and attitudes held by patients, their carers, patient organisations and the general public about health-care professionals and health services. Big changes are already beginning to take place in the way that patients and health professionals relate to one another. The Department of Health and the NHS Executive now actively encourage partnerships between patients and health-care professionals in the delivery of services. New role developments in all professions should start from patients and their needs, which may require revolutions in existing structures, services and even professions. Change will not happen overnight but small adjustments in service delivery can have a vast impact on the quality of life, emotional well-being and self-confidence of both patient and carer.

REFERENCES

Department of Health (DoH) (1990) NHS and Community Care Act. HMSO, London

Department of Health (DoH) (1998) A first-class service. Stationery Office, London

Pharmaceutical Partners UK (PP-UK) (1998) Making partnerships work. Towards best practice in partnerships between the pharmaceutical industry and voluntary health organisations. Hawker, London

World Health Organization (WHO) (1994) Declaration of the promotion of patients' rights in Europe. WHO, Amsterdam

8

A medical perspective

Ann Drury

Introduction

Recognition of the need to review training needs and to eliminate burdensome working practices for junior doctors has been a concern for the medical profession, Government and health-care managers for many years and numerous reports have identified the need to address these issues. This chapter outlines the changes which have been taking place in medical education, in parallel with those in the education and training of nurses and health-care professions (HCPs). The catalyst for changes in medical education was the Department of Health's introduction of the 'New deal on junior doctors' hours' (Department of Health 1991) and the so-called 'Calman report' or, to give it its official title, 'Hospital doctors: training for the future' (Department of Health 1993). The reduction in hours for doctors in training and the changes in medical education will be discussed separately, although as will be seen, they are interlinked and will in time become increasingly interwoven, mirroring the many changes in other health-care professions. Specific examples to illustrate particular points are given from the area of clinical oncology.

'New deal on junior doctors' hours'

Until 1991, when the 'New deal' was brought in, there were no limitations on the hours which doctors in training were expected to, or could be contracted to work. It was not unusual for these doctors to be working anywhere between 80 and 120 hours per week. In addition, as medical science has progressed and the amount of interventions and procedures has increased, the nature of the work on-call for acute admissions of whatever specialty, in 'routine' clinics and for general inpatient care, has also become more intense.

Doctors in training first received overtime payments in 1975 following protracted discussions between the Department of Health and the British Medical Association (BMA). The BMA is the doctors' professional organisation and certificated trade union. A system based on units of medical time (UMTs) was introduced. This was a novel approach to overtime because a UMT equated to 4 hours of work and claims could only be made if more than 2 hours of overtime had been worked. Later this was changed when additional duty hours (ADHs) were introduced and each hour worked was then counted in overtime calculations.

Once the 'New deal' was agreed nationally Regional Task Forces were set up to assist Trusts with establishing how best to implement it throughout England, Wales and Northern Ireland. (Scotland had separate arrangements.) Trusts were visited on a regular basis by Task Forces which were allocated resources from a central fund to create new consultant posts in order to alleviate junior doctors' hours. At that time it was recognised that much of patient care was carried out by pre-registration house officers, senior house officers, registrars and senior registrars, when in fact it would have been more appropriate for an increased total number of consultants to carry out an increased percentage of this care. However, due to the shortage of consultant posts this was not possible and therefore the Department of Health allocated resources to enable Task Forces to create extra consultant posts. The original idea of these posts was that some patient care would be taken from registrars and senior registrars and passed on to consultants, thus releasing registrars and senior registrars from some of their heavy workloads to allow them more time to be taught and reduce the hours they worked.

This was not an easy task. At the outset there was tremendous resistance from many consultants and managers, who felt that the targets set were unachievable. It is interesting that at this stage (i.e. by 1994) the targets were to reduce the hours to 83 contracted which, even at that time, seemed excessive for anyone. Consultant posts were allocated, some staff grade posts were also allocated and slowly a shift could be seen.

The 'New deal' stated that medical education should take place within working hours and should not be an add-on. This was a new concept within medical education. It had always been felt that medical knowledge was gained while practising medicine and that lecture courses and further education were matters which on the whole should take place outside working hours due to heavy service loads and custom and practice. If working 120 hours were considered the norm, one can only wonder how doctors trained in the past ever achieved an adequate level of education in its broadest sense.

Other changes also became necessary in order to reduce working hours. Administrative and support tasks such as filing, bed-finding, chasing X-ray reports, grovelling to X-ray departments in order to obtain X-rays, portering and so on were identified as being inappropriately undertaken by doctors because there was no one else to do them. Shifting these tasks to others was seen as a way of freeing up doctors' time to enable them to concentrate more closely on patient care. In addition it was identified that there were other members of the health-care team who could undertake activities such as phlebotomy, cannulation and the routine administration of intravenous drugs and perform them to a higher and a more consistent level than overworked and inexperienced junior doctors.

The concept of nurses and HCPs working alongside doctors has always been one which has been fully explored and incorporated into the practice of clinical oncology. This may well be related to the origins of the specialty, when clinical oncology came fairly low down the pecking order of allocation for junior medical staff. Therefore, self-reliance within the specialty became the norm, and in order to provide a good service to patients, tasks were shared evenly and new clinical roles were developed.

In order to implement the 'New deal' it became increasingly apparent that major changes in working practices within acute NHS Trusts were required in order to meet the stipulated hours targets. It also became apparent that acute Trusts would be required to work more efficiently and that patient care should be more targeted. So, for example, acute medical admission units were introduced, which greatly reduced the number of patients being admitted randomly throughout hospitals, improved the quality of care and even reduced lengths of stay.

The hours targets set for December 1996 were 56 hours worked, with up to 72 hours on-call. These targets have almost been achieved, albeit 3 years later. With this further reduction in hours, it became even more important that doctors should receive a structured education rather than a haphazard apprenticeship and therefore proper training programmes were required. The 'Calman report' (Department of Health 1993) suggested that medical training should be a much more structured experience which required the way in which training took place to be altered and appropriate training programmes to be set up, or adapted where they were already in place. Implementation of this has taken some years.

'Hospital doctors: training for the future'

The 'Calman report' on postgraduate medical education formed the backbone for the present structure of postgraduate education in medicine in the United Kingdom. The report reviewed the existing arrangements for specialist training and called for changes consistent with European Community (EC) law. It also identified areas for further review and development. The UK was not meeting directives drawn up by the European Commission in 1975. It was felt that there would be an infringement of European law if the UK were not to recognise other member state certificates as being evidence of completion of specialist training. Second, the Commission considered that if the UK certificate, issued for the purposes of the 1975 Medical Directives, was awarded at an intermediate point during postgraduate teaching rather than at its completion, this would have been contrary to the directive. On this basis the UK's position was considered to be unsatisfactory and the Commission decided to initiate proceedings against the UK. The 'Calman report' was then commissioned to review and harmonise UK medical specialist qualifications with those of the rest of Europe.

The report recommended the following:

◆ the introduction of improved training programmes by the end of 1995
◆ the establishment of a single training grade by mid-1995 to replace the career registrar and senior registrar grades
◆ the establishment of regular discussions between the educational bodies and the postgraduate deans as soon as possible
◆ the introduction of a new Certificate of Completion of Specialist Training (CCST). This was to be awarded by the General Medical Council (GMC) on the advice of the appropriate college that a doctor had completed a training programme which met the requirements of the EC directives to a standard compatible with independent practice and conferred eligibility for consideration for appointment to a consultant post.

The report also identified the need for the award of a CCST or equivalent qualification from other EC member states, to be shown on the medical register by the introduction of 'CT' (completion of training) or 'SR' (specialist register) as a specialist indicator, together with the relevant specialty, the year of award and the member state in which the qualification was awarded. The regulator, the GMC, remains responsible for maintaining the register.

The implications of these recommendations for the consultant appointment system were noted, and it was recommended that guidance for Advisory Appointment Committee members should be reconsidered and new guidance incorporating their requirements was issued. For the first time a national quality standard was effectively created for appointments to consultant posts.

The report also considered wider issues such as how the UK input into EC medical legislation and liaison with European colleagues might be better organised. It called for the establishment of improved communication and liaison arrangements, including changes in the membership of the UK delegation to the Advisory Committee on Medical Training (ACMT). The implications for career structure, workforce planning and service provision were also discussed, as was the need for an increase in the number of consultant posts.

Finally, the report noted the need for transitional arrangements during the period of change from one system to another and set out the main strands of action required. It recommended that the changes should be implemented within 2 years of being accepted by ministers and that the Chief Medical Officer should monitor the action being taken forward.

The new training times for medicine set out in the original document provided greater clarity:

◆ 1 year as a pre-registration house officer (PRHO)
◆ 18 months–2 years in general professional training, at senior house officer (SHO) level
◆ 5 years as a specialist registrar (SpR) in the individual's chosen specialty, at the end of which time the doctor concerned would be awarded a CCST.

Many within the medical profession felt that the training could not be achieved in the allotted time (remembering that training to consultant level had taken 10–12 years on average prior to this) and indeed, some specialties have extended the training to 6 years and even longer. Following the acceptance of this report much thought was required to set up programmes to deliver this shortened training adequately.

In 1996 the Department of Health issued 'A guide to the specialist registrar training', known as the 'Orange book'. This was the definitive guide for the training of specialist registrars. It offered guidance for those wishing to enter the grade, those managing it and those providing training programmes. It provided all the information relating to the appointment and employment of this grade of doctor. A second revised edition (DoH 1998) was produced 2 years later which addressed some of the deficits apparent in the first report. As training programmes came into being it was evident that the trainees would need to spend more time being trained and less time providing a service. This in turn increased pressures on NHS Trusts to find alternative ways of delivering services.

The responsibility for doctors in training is delegated to the postgraduate dean. It is a heavy burden and as more directives are issued it becomes increasingly complex. The responsibility was originally merely supervisory but there is now financial responsibility too. In recognition of the training element received from the Trusts by SHOs and SpRs the postgraduate medical dean passes on to Trusts 50% of the trainee's basic salary at SHO and SpR level and 100% at PRHO level (known as MADEL – Medical and Dental Educational Levy – funding). The funding of all overtime payments is the responsibility of individual Trusts.

Record of In-Training Assessment (RITA)

During SpR training, yearly assessment takes place. This has been a significant change for medical education. Since the full implementation of SpR training these assessments have become more structured and accepted by trainers and trainees as both essential and helpful. The process is overseen by the postgraduate deanery and guidelines as to how this should take place are issued by each regional deanery, which sets out the role of the SpR trainer, the Trust.

The role of the Trust is to ensure that structures are in place to deliver the following for all trainees:

◆ quality induction
◆ clearly defined supervisory arrangements, identified educational supervisors and adequate clinical supervision
◆ objective-setting within a short period of taking up post or moving to a different team/firm, appraisal and regular opportunities for professional conversations to take place
◆ agreed educational plans between the trainee and the educational supervisor
◆ regular assessment of competence based on objective criteria and handled in a transparent manner with substantiated evidence of poor performance and conduct, where necessary
◆ where necessary, the support to deliver defined remedial training
◆ ensuring that clinical responsibility is tailored to a realistic assessment of the trainees' competence
◆ the availability of a mentor if requested by individual trainees
◆ pastoral support for doctors in trouble.

The function of the Record of In-Training Assessment (RITA) is:

◆ to record and manage trainees' progress towards their training goal and through the SpR grade

◆ to provide a mechanism which reviews and encourages open and fair assessment
◆ to provide a framework to link the responsibilities for assessment and review of progress, between the Royal Colleges (and Faculties) to those of the postgraduate deans
◆ to enable assessment of out-of-programme clinical work
◆ to provide a final statement of the trainee's successful completion of the training programme.

This is not in itself a means of assessment but a review of progress based on the in-placement assessment according to Royal College/Faculty rules.

Pre-registration house officers (PRHOs)

The training of doctors following qualification from medical school in their pre-registration year, i.e. prior to full registration with the GMC, was set out and updated in the GMC's recommendations on general clinical training (1997a). Unfortunately subsequent visits and interviews with PRHOs, clinical tutors, educational supervisors and postgraduate deans demonstrated that the quality of training continued to vary across the country and new standards were set out in an attempt to bring all posts up to the standard of the best.

These latest recommendations are set out in the 'New doctor' published by the GMC (1997b) and are now being implemented. One of the key themes concerns the requirement to support PRHOs and facilitate their learning. It stresses the requirement for supervision by a fully trained specialist while PRHOs are learning to become doctors by providing a service and emphasises the need for due regard to their educational needs. Regular inspection of the PRHO posts is carried out by the relevant university and encompassed within this is a requirement that these posts have hours and conditions of work which are within the 'New deal' guidelines. Also contained within the document is an important pointer for the future of medical training and practice in the recognition of the role of other professions in the process of collaborative learning and assessment:

> Nurses and other non-medical staff are an important source of information, support and guidance for PRHOs as they make the transition from medical student to practising professional. Their views on the clinical progress being made by PRHOs will be invaluable to educational supervisors and they should also alert supervisors to any shortcomings in PRHO performance. Some health care professionals have particular skills to impart to PRHOs, for example, the expertise which Macmillan nurses have in palliative care, and such multidisciplinary education/learning opportunities are to be encouraged. (GMC 1997b)

This is a great leap forward in medical education and recognises the fact that throwing doctors in at the deep end, as was once the case, is no longer a safe or appropriate way to train and retain doctors in the future.

Senior house officers (SHOs)

Senior house officers still do not have a formal structure of training like PRHOs and SpRs. They have been and are still regarded by many as the 'lost tribe' (British Medical Association 1998). The educational content of these posts is overseen by either the dean of general practice if the post is recognised for general practice vocational training (GPVT), or the Royal College of that particular specialty, or both. The training, however, is less structured but considerable effort is being exerted at present to rectify this situation. The GMC published a booklet similar to that pertaining to PRHOs which sets out the duties and training objectives of SHOs (GMC 1998). It encourages high-quality patient care through education and training and sets out the responsibilities of the postgraduate deans, director of postgraduate general practice education, associate deans and clinical tutors, Health Authorities and NHS Trusts and all others involved in training and supervision.

Some really encouraging content is that:

> The views of nurses and other health care professionals about the clinical progress being made by SHOs will be invaluable to the trainees and their educational supervisors. Problems should be discussed with trainees and, if these persist, educational supervisors should be alerted. Other health care professionals may also have particular skills to impart to SHOs, and such inter-professional educational and learning opportunities should be encouraged. (GMC 1998: para 62)

One of the difficulties which is beginning to be recognised is the over-provision of SHOs in relation to the number of SpR posts available. The number of SHOs was initially expanded as part of meeting the early 'New deal' targets. The number of potential consultant vacancies that are estimated to arise regulates the number of SpR posts. A committee called the Specialist Workforce Advisory Group (SWAG) calculates these numbers. These numbers take into account the potential increased requirement in consultant numbers from either an expansion in service in a certain specialty (including retirements), as well as any potential for reduction. This is not an easy calculation and cannot in all fairness take account of factors as yet unknown. It does, however, need to take into account changing working practices in nursing and HCPs. For example, in clinical oncology the opportunity for expanding the role of therapeutic radiographers should be taken into account, especially with regard to their potential role in prescribing palliative treatments, simple treatments and running their own on-treatment clinics (School of Health and Related Research 1999). Maintaining a balance of the right skills within the health workforce is a complex process; at present there are far more SHO posts than there are SpR posts and a bottleneck to career progression is therefore being created. Yet the growing demands of the service are likely to require more doctors (Parliamentary Select Committee on Health 1999). Unless this situation is addressed quickly there will be many disillusioned doctors.

Sharing of care

The sharing of patient care with nurses and HCPs is not a new concept in many specialties. If clinical oncology/medical oncology is taken as an example, there has been for very many years a very close working relationship between doctors, nurses, radiographers, social workers, physiotherapists, occupational therapists and others.

This working relationship may in part be historical. As previously mentioned, at the outset clinical oncology was a Cinderella specialty and did not attract as many trainees as other specialties such as surgery and medicine. Teamwork therefore became the only way of delivering a good-quality service. Nurses and others were and are encouraged to become experts in their field, their knowledge and expertise is acknowledged and respected and this forms the basis for strong team working. This is not to say that there are not barriers to joint working. One of the barriers is the way in which the pre-clinical medical education of doctors is organised. Doctors in the main are trained separately from nurses and HCPs and many can have difficulties (probably as a result of this) in working with and being taught by the other health professions. There are now, however, several universities which are undertaking a more collaborative approach to training by implementing joint training and shared learning opportunities pre- and post-registration for the health professions where relevant. This should foster a more open approach to joint working in the future. It is evident that there is a huge scope for further collaborative practice between all the health-care professions as the demarcation between them becomes increasingly less relevant. These changes can only be for the good as they provide opportunities for those who wish to avail themselves of the potential to expand their roles by taking on more advanced care, but only if they are integrated into the team.

The definition of team working is not always well understood, and it is important to remember that just as in a football team different members bring different qualities and expertise to the team. Those who work in different aspects of the patient's care can bring their own perspectives to that care. This is especially so with nurses in oncology, who see patients holistically and in many respects are more able to judge their physical and emotional needs. They spend more time with patients talking to them about everyday occurrences, their families, their employment and their homes. It is often nurses who are first to spot from clues such as a change in the patient's appearance how things are progressing or not and therefore a multidisciplinary perspective is key in any discussion of the patient's management.

Change in service patterns

Changes in patterns of service provision have meant that consultants need to take a more hands-on approach, though in fairness the majority had already begun to do so and the stress imposed on them cannot be underestimated in this exercise (KPMG 1997, 1998). Consultants are now required to do more teaching as well as provide more service and they feel the squeeze very keenly. To some extent providing extra consultant posts has helped but these numbers are not huge. Throughout the UK the total allocation of new consultants was approximately 200–250 new posts.

Through the work of 'New deal', Task Forces in each NHS region have had their attention drawn to a variety of innovative working practices such as those associated with cardiac surgery in Oxford. One cardiac surgeon implemented the introduction of a nurse who was trained as a 'Surgeon's assistant'. This role entailed a wide range of duties which included taking the vein graft from the patient's leg, prior to bypass surgery. This new role demonstrated that others outside the medical profession could carry out patient care at a high level and is often cited as an example to persuade doctors that their workload can be shared with their colleagues in nursing and the HCPs. It also demonstrated that patients could indeed receive even better quality and continuity of care if good team working was implemented. It has to be said that at the outset this change in working practices met considerable opposition from some sectors of the medical profession. This was because many doctors saw these changes as being detrimental to patient care, or were reluctant to accept that changes in their practice could result in a better pattern of care.

Yet, as the pace of change in medicine becomes ever more rapid, continuing medical education is becoming increasingly necessary if doctors are to keep up with the changes which are evolving. At present it is not a requirement for maintenance on the Specialist Register that continuing medical education is recorded and documented. The Bristol cases of child deaths following cardiac surgery and other notable cases have highlighted the need for re-accreditation and the methods to implement this are presently being investigated. It should, however, be remembered that it is the responsibility of all medical practitioners to keep abreast of new advances within their practice, and to have an awareness of their own limitations and to put this into practice.

Future perspectives

The training and future practice of the medical profession will be required to alter if it is to cope with the challenges that lie ahead. Changes have already taken place, but in order to keep pace with the requirements of the present and the future a far more open attitude to different ways of providing care will need to be adopted.

The number of students entering medical school is set to rise by 1000 per annum, giving a yearly intake of 6000. However, even this increase will not be sufficient to allow the profession to continue along its present path. There will need to be many more nurses and HCPs trained to a higher level, taking on more responsibility and therefore having a far greater say in the way in which patient care is provided.

Another aspect which will force change on practice is the introduction of the 48-hour week for doctors in training. (This restriction already applies to nurses, HCPs and non-training grade doctors.) There will be fewer doctors available and therefore this will act as a further catalyst for change.

A 'higher level of practice' has already begun to be recognised within the nursing profession with the creation of 'nurse consultants' who are confident enough to expand their roles. Other higher levels of practice are beginning to be implemented – for example, in radiography, where diagnostic radiographers in one teaching hospital are starting to undertake angiography.

It is to be hoped that medicine as a whole can move forward by joint working and learning with all those involved in patient care. This will require a far more open attitude than presently prevails within the higher echelons of the medical profession. Let us hope, however, that future care will be delivered by a genuine team approach with greater understanding of each other's roles and contribution.

REFERENCES

British Medical Association (BMA) (1998) The future of the SHO grade: report of the Junior Doctors Committee Working Party in SHO Training. BMA, London
Department of Health (DoH) (1991) New deal on junior doctors' hours. HMSO, London
Department of Health (1993) Hospital doctors: training for the future. Report of the Working Group on Specialist Medical Training. Department of Health, London (Chair Sir K Calman)
Department of Health (DoH) (1998) A guide to the specialist registrar training, 2nd edn. Stationery Office, London

School of Health and Related Research (SCHARR) (1999) Exploring new roles in practice. SCHARR, University of Sheffield, Sheffield

General Medical Council (GMC) (1997a) Protecting patients, guiding doctors. GMC, London

General Medical Council (GMC) (1997b) The new doctor. GMC, London

General Medical Council (GMC) (1998) The early years. GMC, London

KPMG (1997) Research into changes in the work of consultants. Office of Manpower Economics, London

KPMG (1998) Aspects of the workload of hospital consultants. Office of Manpower Economics, London

Parliamentary Select Committee on Health (1999) Third report: future NHS staffing requirements. Stationery Office, London

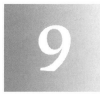

9

Evaluating new role development

Debra Humphris   Abigail Masterson

Introduction

'The new NHS: modern, dependable' (Department of Health 1997) sets out a

10-year modernisation strategy for the UK health service. Key supplementary papers outlining the detail of this modernisation programme, which have direct relevance for the evaluation of new role developments, include 'A first-class service', 'Working together', 'Information for health', 'Saving lives' and the existing research and development strategy, 'Research for health'.

'A first-class service' (Department of Health 1998) focuses on improving the quality of patient care. It introduces for the time ever a statutory duty of quality, which will apply to all NHS organisations in the form of clinical governance. Clinical governance is defined as 'a framework through which all NHS organisations are accountable for continuously improving the quality of their services and safeguarding high standards of care by creating an environment in which excellence in clinical care will flourish'.

One of the key aims of 'Working together' (NHS Executive 1999) is to ensure a quality workforce in the right numbers, with the right skills and diversity and organised in the right way to deliver the Government's service objectives for health and social care. The evolution of work roles within health care is both desirable and inevitable. Successful patient-centred change is dependent upon holistic evaluation benefiting from a variety of perspectives. To date, many of these new role developments have lacked rigorous evaluation (School of Health and Related Research 1997). This is in part due to the ad hoc nature of the developments themselves, their route of funding, and the often expedient nature of their implementation. Developing a wider evaluative culture within health-care delivery will depend upon fully evaluating human resource changes as well as changes in interventions and practices. At the time of writing the Department of Health (England) had commenced a process of tendering for such evaluations. The aim of this initiative is to deliver research which will contribute significantly to the evidence base for human resource policies and practice, and underpin the human resources framework set out in 'Working together'. Funds of around £2.5 million have been made available for this programme of research.

'Information for health' (NHS Executive 1998) underpins the objectives and targets of Health Improvement Programmes, and in particular will facilitate integrated working across organisations and care settings. It is not merely concerned with the implementation of information systems; through that investment it aims to facilitate a range of benefits such as multiprofessional, multi-agency needs assessment, care planning, provision and monitoring. However, information management and technology investment will require organisational and cultural shifts if the necessary changes in working practices are to be realised. Without these changes this investment will be wasted. For example, the 'development of the potential of telemedicine can facilitate new ways of delivering health care. But this requires changes in attitude and behaviour and a willingness of professionals to communicate with each other and across professional and organisational boundaries.

One specific aspect of 'Saving Lives' (Department of Health 1999) illustrates perfectly the transfer of technological understanding and skill to the wider public in order to promote health. The emphasis on teaching resuscitation skills and making available equipment such as defibrillators in public places illustrates how skills that used to be confined to health-care professionals in critical care environments are being disseminated and shared for the wider public good.

'Research for Health' (DoH 1991) sets out the aim of developing a 'knowledge-based service', and states that therefore any new role development logically requires evaluation before expansion, an element which has been lacking in many areas. We will now consider which approaches can be used most appropriately to evaluate the impact of new clinical roles upon services, patients and the professions.

Whose perspective to include

Any evaluation of a new role will need to include a range of perspectives, not just those of the postholder and those who have supported the development. No single change in a system can occur in isolation, but will have a ripple effect upon many other players within that context. Therefore multiple perspectives should be considered when undertaking an evaluation.

Consumers

The perspective of the consumers of a service is often overlooked, but is key to robust evaluation of service developments. There are undeniably challenges involved in accessing and ascertaining this perspective but ultimately consumers are the guardians of legitimacy. Too often service developments are not explained to consumers, never mind their views sought on the appropriateness, efficiency and effectiveness of changes. As Funnell makes clear in Chapter 7 of this book, too often the consumer perspective is engaged merely to provide legitimacy to a professionally led development, rather than consumer views being sought prior to the decision-making process about the direction of travel. Signs of change are becoming evident as consumer organisations are increasingly funding new role developments and their evaluation. For example, the British Heart Foundation is engaged in fundraising for, and the employment and evaluation of specialist nursing, occupational therapy and physiotherapy roles. Engaging the consumer perspective within the process of evaluation is not easy; there are numerous considerations and complexities, for which advice can be sought from bodies such as the College of Health, a health consumer campaigning organisation. The involvement of consumers is no longer a luxury but a necessity.

Practitioners

The challenge of the evaluative process for practitioners often has to be set alongside the demands of the role itself. Being responsible for the delivery of a service and its evaluation can create paradoxical demands. First of all the immediacy of service delivery can tend to crowd out the time needed for critical reflection. Second, it is difficult for practitioners to escape from the detail of their practice and adopt a broader objective view of their contribution to the service as an entirety. Undertaking an evaluation is itself a complex and difficult task. One of the key dilemmas that practitioners in new roles face is the need to justify their existence, which may lead them to construct a defence for the continuation of the post rather than an objective evaluation of its service contribution. For example, nurse specialists often argue that an indicator of their success would be that they have worked themselves out of their job. However, there is little evidence that this has ever happened. Practitioners are therefore faced with the dilemmas of whether they should undertake their own evaluations, and how they can develop the skills necessary to do that. Practitioners quite rightly are usually appointed to such posts for their clinical skills rather than their evaluative expertise. However, this does not negate the need to undertake evaluation of new roles; it requires instead that it should occur as part of a wider workforce evaluation, and be undertaken by those with the appropriate skills.

Researchers

The relationship between the research community and the health service has come under increasing scrutiny. Research teams are still mainly based in higher education institutions (HEIs) in unidisciplinary teams. The focus in many HEIs is on undertaking research that will count towards the Research Assessment Exercise (RAE). The RAE is a quality 'league table' where academic outputs in relation to research and the development of the knowledge base of a discipline are judged in terms of their significance nationally and internationally. The RAE has considerable significance for HEIs in relation to their funding and the profile of the organisation. Success in the RAE therefore affects recruitment of students and staff. Effective evaluation of health service delivery often requires a multidisciplinary perspective and draws on a variety of scientific traditions. Commentators such as Becher (1989) have noted that within HEIs unidisciplinary working predominates. The RAE has so far further encouraged this unidisciplinary focus as individual departments within organisations are encouraged to compete for the highest rating. Pure research is more highly valued than applied, little value is placed on multiprofessional research and scant attention is paid to the social utility of the findings. General underfunding of the university sector has also necessitated them making prohibitive charges (anything from 40–60% is common) for 'overheads', which may place the cost of an evaluation beyond the budget of many service providers. Since the identification of health service evaluation as a new discipline – health service research, and the establishment of a Service Delivery and Organisation Programme within the NHS research and development structure – dedicated funding is becoming available and therefore interest and flexibility from the research community may increase.

Human resource staff

Since its inception the NHS has lacked a strategic focus on workforce planning in relation to health-care and service need. Workforce planning has been split across a variety of bodies, most of which have operated in isolation and not necessarily in concert with each other. For example, medical workforce planning has to date been separate from that of nurses and health-care professions (HCPs), with whom such staff work in clinical teams. Professionals working in human resources have tended to be restricted to the recruitment and retention of staff within predetermined parameters, rather than being enabled to consider the workforce as a whole. For example, the funding and staffing of human resource professionals themselves has been strictly separated into medical and non-medical. Likewise the purchasing of education for initial professional preparation and post-registration education remains separate and controlled by different bodies. Recent high-level and influential reports such as 'The future of the healthcare workforce' (Health Services Management Unit 1996) and 'The workforce and training implications of the Calman/Hine cancer report' (The Cancer Collaboration 1997) have highlighted these anomalies (see Chapter 8). All of this serves to indicate the urgent need for human resource professionals to be more actively involved in the evaluation of all clinical roles, as part of fostering the evaluative culture that clinical governance will demand.

Managers

Managers have traditionally focused on 'getting the job done', often to the neglect of critical reflection upon the effectiveness of changes to roles. Pressures to introduce new roles have often come from forces beyond the managers' direct control, and when faced with the opportunity to appoint extra staff expedience often wins over a broader attention to longer-term effectiveness. In a similar way to human resource staff, managers have not always been fully engaged in debates about the importance of evaluation, and therefore may lack the skills or resources to support such work. Equally, the organisation itself may have lacked an evaluative ethic in terms of new role developments, and may have focused mainly on the audit of activity as a measure of productivity. Managers need to be involved in evaluations as they can bring a broader service perspective than the practitioner, and can in turn apply that learning to future service changes. In addition, two of the factors that inhibit practitioners from being involved in evaluation are time and resources, and managers can have an appreciation of and an influence over both of these.

Other team members

The implementation of any new role will have implications for the wider system of working, and such posts cannot be considered in isolation. It is therefore imperative to map the terrain in terms of other practitioners within the team when attempting to understand and evaluate the impact of changes in clinical roles. A small change in one role may result in fundamental questions being raised for other practitioners. For example, the role of the diabetes nurse specialist often includes the provision of dietary advice; if this support is sufficient to meet the needs of the patient, it in turn raises questions regarding the contribution of dieticians to the care of this client group. Where new roles are the result of substitution, such as neonatal nurse practitioners substituting for junior doctors in special care baby units, and rheumatology practitioners who are often physiotherapists or occupational therapists substituting for junior doctors in the outpatient care of people with long-term rheumatological conditions, the need for a whole team approach to deciding on appropriate comparators is paramount. The opportunity afforded by involvement in a 'whole system' approach can also enable a greater shared understanding of the process and outcome of evaluation.

How to go about an evaluation

When undertaking an evaluation there are a number of factors to be considered at the planning stage. This list is by no means exhaustive, but should provide you with some indication of the complexities that need to be considered.

Context

This includes issues about the location, place and time in which an evaluation is taking place. One of the things that helps make sense of smaller-scale evaluations and enhances the potential generalisability of the lessons learned is a full description of the context. For example, organisational charts, reporting arrangements, funding sources, the nature of the organisation's business, geographical location, workforce stability and turnover, service uptake and use, and the position of the development in relation to business planning cycles are key for others in determining the appropriateness or otherwise of such developments in their own context.

Supporters and detractors

Evaluation is always undertaken within the 'political' context of the setting. There will be a range of views on the activity and its subject, only some of which will be supportive. What remains vital to the evaluative process is that the views of both supporters and detractors are recognised, and taken into account in a balanced and rigorous way.

Funding resources

In an ideal world the funding for new role developments would include an evaluative component. Currently this is rarely the case, however. Often external funding must be sought to support evaluation. Funding agencies will often have strict criteria for awarding grants, which may automatically exclude small-scale service development. Writing project grant proposals demands a specialist range of skills, which practitioners and managers may not possess, and so partnership with an HEI may be necessary. Budgetary constraints often make it difficult for NHS organisations to support systematic evaluation activity. However, as the importance of workforce evaluation becomes more evident it may well be that more resources will be identified for this purpose.

Method

It is impossible to give a definitive methodological approach because by necessity each new role is unique to its context and may require different methodological considerations. However, there are some key principles which should govern all evaluative activity. From the outset it is important to be clear about the question, to ensure that the method selected is appropriate to address the question, and that the method is applied rigorously. Most evaluations fail because insufficient attention is paid to clarifying the question. If this preparation isn't undertaken the wrong data may be collected; this will not provide the information needed and may lead to erroneous conclusions being drawn.

A useful planning guide is offered by St Leger et al (1992), which sets out five critical points in planning an evaluative study:

◆ setting objectives
◆ selecting a study design
◆ organising data collection
◆ developing protocols
◆ setting up channels of communication.

Clarifying the question

Clarifying the question is the hardest part of the evaluative process and therefore is the one worth spending most time on. The purpose of an evaluation is to make a judgement about the extent to which a new role has achieved its goals. Therefore all those parties who have an interest in the process and outcome should be involved in framing the question. In some circumstances the scale and scope of the evaluation will constrain what it is possible to do. Therefore the quest for clarity must be combined with realism. This may in turn mean that some of the objectives stakeholders would like to achieve may not be possible.

If this is a role that has been put in place without a clear job description or role definition it is at this stage that the importance of those elements becomes most evident. Without a job description/tight role definition it will be difficult to find appropriate standards, benchmarks or indices of comparison to measure against. Similarly, if the evaluation is being carried out retrospectively and the role itself has evolved this can undermine attempts to clarify a meaningful measurement of impact.

Unless the question is clear the wrong data may well be collected and time and resources wasted. Clarifying the question will also affect the method chosen. To illustrate the impact of these choices we offer a case study in Box 9.1.

Design

The design of any evaluation will have to take into account the aims and objectives, timescale and resources, and the degree of rigour required.

Aims and objectives

There are two main research approaches or paradigms in research. These are commonly referred to quantitative and qualitative approaches. Broadly, quantitative approaches focus on measurement whereas qualitative approaches

Box 9.1 A case study

Jackie is a therapeutic radiographer working in a large teaching hospital which is a regional cancer centre. She noticed that women attending for radiotherapy appeared not to be having their needs for information and psychological support met at the time of therapy. She approached her manager with a view to expanding her role to offer this kind of support. Her manager agreed that Jackie could increase her appointment times in order to spend more time with the women giving information and offering advice and support. Increasing pressure on the manager's budget forced her to question the effectiveness of this additional expenditure. The initial feedback from women accessing the service had seemed favourable. The manager was reluctant to cut the service simply because of budget pressures and therefore Jackie was given the responsibility of justifying this role expansion.

Evaluation is concerned with assessing whether or not a service or intervention achieves its goals. In the case study outlined there are several questions that an evaluation could address. For example, a fundamental question would be: Does the service work? That is, as a result of Jackie spending time 'counselling' women, were those women more informed about their treatment? The manager might want to identify whether the service was efficient in terms of making best use of existing resources and would therefore ask whether the way that Jackie was delivering the service was efficient. In other words, were there other ways in which the women could have gained the same information and support from other sources? From the women's point of view the question of Jackie's competence to undertake this additional role might be important to their overall satisfaction with the service offered. Equity might also be a key issue here. Did all women receive the enhanced service or only those who saw Jackie? Colleagues might want to know about the knock-on effect of the reduction in Jackie's workload in terms of the number of radiography treatments delivered for the rest of the department.

Think point
Whilst all of these questions are of interest to different stakeholders in the evaluation process the resource constraints of a localised evaluation will necessitate that only one or two of these questions can be addressed in the evaluation. This immediately illustrates the importance of the unanswered questions in forming a comprehensive evaluation of a new role development. From this example you may want to reflect on which questions you feel should be selected and why.

focus on meaning. From the outset it is important that careful consideration is given to selecting the appropriate approach to address the objectives of the proposed evaluation. Taking the case study described earlier, workload is amenable to quantitative measurement and can be investigated using routinely collected data such as number of staff hours available, number of patients seen, doses administered and treatment duration. However, if patient satisfaction were the focus of the evaluation then data would need to be collected on the patient experience. This would involve gathering subjective judgements from the women of the service they received. This data could be collected using interviews, focus groups or questionnaires. Every woman's construction of satisfaction is personal and wholly valid and will not therefore be amenable to straightforward measurement or comparison. However, when analysed rigorously, qualitative data of this sort would provide an extremely rich source of information about the women's satisfaction with the service. Depending on the aim of the evaluation the design of the study will vary and the key evaluation question should dictate the method selected. Increasingly both meaning and measurement are recognised as having an important place in the overall evaluation of services. Evaluation designs are beginning to reflect this by drawing upon both research traditions (Goodwin & Goodwin 1984, Inui 1996).

Timescale and resources

Timescale and resources may both constrain evaluation designs and conversely offer opportunities. Timescales may be imposed internally or externally. Evaluation designs will also dictate the time required to complete the evaluation. For example, if an evaluation required 20 patients attending a new clinic to be interviewed and every tenth patient was to be selected Jackie would need to have treated 200 people in order to have met her sampling requirements. There may also be a number of factors such as holidays, medical staff leave and so on that would lead to a variation in referral rates and could also have a delaying effect on Jackie seeing sufficient patients. Often an external funder will dictate the timescale within which the evaluation is completed. For example, a grant application may require that the work is completed within 1 year but variations in referral rates and over-optimistic judgements about sample size may lead an evaluation to fail to meet the timescale.

No matter how many of the questions in the case study described above it would be interesting to address, there has to be a balance between what is possible and what is desirable within the resources available. Even when resources are limited this should not compromise rigour but should focus the evaluator's minds as to how best to construct an appropriate design. Take, for example, the question raised in the case study about the effectiveness of Jackie's counselling intervention: Does the service work? That is, as a result of Jackie spending time 'counselling' women, were the women more informed about their treatment? In order to address this question properly the design of an evaluation may need to include a way of measuring the effect of Jackie's intervention against some comparison which may include no intervention. To do this in an effective way would require a trial in which the intervention was controlled and the individuals receiving it were randomly allocated to Jackie or other groups. This would enable measurement of the different forms of intervention against one another. For example, there might be three groups established: Jackie, a nurse providing similar counselling and no extra support. This type of design is known as a randomised controlled trial. Establishing such a trial would require considerable resources, ethical approval and the consent of the women to participate. This may be beyond the capability and capacity available within Jackie's organisation and might require external support. The lack of local resources to address this issue does not make the question any less important but does raise considerable concerns about the extent to which we know if local changes in service are effective. Jackie's aspirations and desires may have been formed with the best intentions but increasingly best intentions will be insufficient to guide service development in establishing new roles.

The evaluation capability and capacity within organisations will influence how much of this work can be undertaken internally. Building the capability of staff who can undertake or contribute to such activity will be important within the wider framework of clinical governance.

Rigour

Rigour is a requirement of all evaluations but the means of ensuring rigour will vary depending on the broad evaluation approach taken. Mays & Pope (1995) have developed a useful checklist in relation to assessing rigour in qualitative research, which we have amended to reflect rigour in qualitative evaluation designs:

◆ Were the approach adopted and the methods used made explicit?
◆ Was the context of the evaluation clearly described?
◆ Was the sampling strategy clearly described and justified?
◆ Did the sampling include a diverse range of individuals and settings, if appropriate, in order to enhance the generalisability of the analysis?
◆ Was the data collection clearly described in detail?
◆ Were the procedures for analysis clearly described and justified?
◆ Can an independent investigator inspect the evaluation material and the procedure for its analysis?
◆ Were a variety of methods used to reflect a range of perspectives within the analysis?

◆ Was enough of the raw data (e.g. transcript and interviews) presented in a systematic fashion to convince the reader that the interpretation of the evaluator was based on the evidence?

There are numerous checklists within the literature that attempt to provide a framework of questions to guide a reader's critical appraisal of papers and reports. The framework set out in Table 9.1, which we have developed from Benton & Cormack (1996), can help you to consider the rigour of any quantitative evaluation.

Table 9.1 Framework for considering rigour in quantitative evaluations

Heading	Question to be asked
Introduction	Is the problem clearly identified? Is a rationale for undertaking the study stated? Are the limitations of the study clearly stated? Is the source of funding for the study identified?
Literature review	Is the literature up to date? Does the literature review identify the underlying theoretical framework(s)? Does the literature review present a balanced evaluation of material both supporting and challenging the position being proposed? Does the literature clearly identify the need for the evaluation proposed? Are all the important and relevant references included?
The hypothesis	Does the study use an experimental approach? Is the hypothesis capable of being tested? Is the hypothesis unambiguous?
Operational definitions	Are all terms used clearly defined?
Methodology	Does the methodology section clearly state the evaluation approach used? Is the method appropriate to the problem? Are the strengths and weaknesses of the chosen approach stated?
Subjects	Are the subjects clearly identified?
Sample selection	Is the sample selection approach congruent with the method to be used? Is the approach to sample selection clearly stated? Is the sample size clearly stated?

Table 9.1 *(cont'd)*

Heading	Question to be asked
Data collection	Are all the data collection procedures adequately described? Have the validity and reliability of any instruments or questionnaires been clearly stated?
Ethical considerations	If the study involves human subjects has the ethical committee granted approval? Has informed consent been sought? Is confidentiality assured? Is anonymity guaranteed?
Results	Are all the results presented? Are the results clearly presented? Are the results internally consistent? Is sufficient detail given to enable the reader to judge how much confidence can be placed in the findings?
Data analysis	Is the approach appropriate to the type of data collected? Is any statistical analysis correctly performed? Is there sufficient analysis to determine whether 'significant differences' are not attributable to variation in other relevant variables? Is complete information (test value, df and p) reported?
Discussion	Is the discussion balanced? Does the discussion draw upon previous research? Are the weaknesses/limitations of the study acknowledged? Are the implications for practice, research, management and policy-making discussed?
Conclusion	Are the conclusions supported by the results obtained?
Recommendations	Do the recommendations relate to the conclusions drawn? Do the recommendations suggest further areas for research/evaluation? Do the recommendations identify how any weaknesses in the study design could be avoided in future research/evaluation?

Locking in the learning

As Palmer has already noted in Chapter 4 of this book the value of learning through experience and critical reflection should not be underestimated. Conducting a rigorous evaluation of any new role will result not only in the direct learning of the outcome of the evaluation but will also provide a source of considerable learning for those who have been involved in the evaluative process. Learning from such experiences generates knowledge, which can be directly supportive to the organisation's future attempts at role evaluation. For example, if a health-care team has been involved in evaluating a new role development it may think differently when it develops roles in the future. It can also be used as a source of support to other teams within the organisation who may be struggling with similar evaluative challenges. Much of this form of knowledge is often referred to as tacit knowledge, which Polyani (1958) described as a set of common-sense non-articulated understandings, through which we make sense of our world. Increasingly these common-sense understandings will enable a more evaluative approach to changes in service delivery. Practitioners and organisations will need to utilise systematically the 'know-how' that is developed about and through evaluation.

Links to organisational human resource strategy

In order to deliver on the government targets set out in 'Working together' (Department of Health, 1999) an integrated programme of human resource management is to be put in place, the third strategic aim of which is to 'address the management capacity and capability to deliver this agenda for change'. Such capacity and capability will require significant investment in evaluation skills as part of establishing a broader evaluative culture within the NHS. Learning from rigorously conducted evaluation of new roles provides a useful starting point from which to build. Human resource strategies within NHS organisations can be a fundamental part of evolving a workforce that reflects patients' needs rather than professional aspirations.

A commitment to build evidence-based services has to be taken on board by clinicians, managers and human resource professionals alike. This may sometimes place human resource professionals at odds with their clinical colleagues when realistic judgements have to be made about the composition and numbers of the future health-care workforce. Many of the new role developments that have emerged could be found lacking in terms of evidence of their effectiveness. For example, the nursing literature is replete with glowing anecdotal and descriptive accounts of new role developments. This is despite a paucity of sound evaluations of such developments. Similarly, the publication of 'The future of the healthcare workforce' (Health Services Management Unit 1996), which advocated radical changes to the composition of the workforce, was met with howls of outrage by the professions who saw it as an attack upon their relative roles and status. By encouraging a more rigorous approach to human resource evaluation it is likely that many of the established vested interests will experience increased discomfort from such work. It is nevertheless foolish for such professionals to advocate evidence-based practice and yet not expect the same discipline and rigour to be applied to all aspects of health care.

Conclusion

There are, of course, always consequences of evaluation. If you ask the questions you have to be able to deal with the answers. For example, in the case study above the outcome might have been that Jackie's intervention was no more effective than no intervention, i.e. that the role had not achieved what it was designed to do. The consequence of this should be that the service is stopped and for Jackie this is likely to be a very uncomfortable decision which would require courage to enact. Yet it would be inappropriate to continue with a role development which was not shown to be any more effective than the existing service. Evaluation is not a luxury but a necessity of responsible role development. Without it resources and energy are wasted, and the opportunities for learning are lost to the organisation.

Evaluation brings many challenges but in the future we should not be creating new roles without a comprehensive and systematic evaluation process. The present government's commitment to investing in the research and development skills of health care professionals is clear. So whilst new roles will constantly be needed so too will there be a requirement for robust and rigorous evaluation of such developments. Partnerships consisting of researchers, human resource staff, managers, consumers and practitioners can draw out the practical and cost-effective implications of such evaluations for future workforce and service development.

REFERENCES

Becher T (1989) Academic tribes and territories: intellectual enquiry and the cultures of disciplines. Society for Research into Higher Education and the Open University Press, Milton Keynes

Benton D C, Cormack D F S (1996) Reviewing and evaluating the literature. In Cormack D F S (ed) The research process in nursing, 3rd edn. Blackwell Science, Oxford

Department of Health (1991) Research for health. Stationery Office, London

Department of Health (1997) The new NHS: modern, dependable. Stationery Office, London (Cm 3807)

Department of Health (1998) A first-class service: quality in the new NHS. Department of Health, London

Department of Health (1999) Saving lives: our healthier nation. Stationery Office, London

Goodwin L D, Goodwin W L (1984) Qualitative vs quantitative research or qualitative and quantitative research? Nursing Research 33(6):378–380

Health Services Management Unit (1996) The future healthcare workforce. University of Manchester, Manchester

Inui T S (1996) The virtue of qualitative and quantitative research. Annals of Internal Medicine 125(9):770–771

Mays N, Pope C (1995) Rigour and qualitative research. British Medical Journal 311:109–112

NHS Executive (1998) Information for health: an information strategy for the modern NHS 1998–2005. A national strategy for local implementation. NHSE, Leeds

NHS Executive (1999) Working together – securing a quality workforce for the NHS. Health Service Circular 79

Polanyi M (1958) Personal knowledge. University of Chicago, Chicago

School of Health and Related Research (SCHARR) (1997) The ENRiP database. SCHARR, University of Sheffield, Sheffield

St Leger A S (1992) Evaluating health services' effectiveness. Open University Press, Milton Keynes

The Cancer Collaboration (1997) The workforce and training implications of the Calman/Hine cancer report. Pharmaceutical Alliance in Cancer Care

10

New role development
Taking a strategic approach

Abigail Masterson   Debra Humphris

Introduction

Changes in health policy such as the shift towards a primary care-led National Health Service (NHS), community care for people with mental health problems, the increased emphasis on women-centred midwifery services, technological advances and increases in scientific knowledge demand that the health-care professions develop in new ways. Changes in the health-care workforce are both the product and consequence of numerous internal and external pressures. The effect of these changes over time will result in the emergence of new clinical roles and the redundancy of others. There is an ongoing need for all of the stakeholders in health care to review the skills and knowledge that are needed to deliver services. For successful service development there should be a continual process of co-evolution between the pressures that shape health care and the workforce needed to deliver it.

Boundaries between the professions have always been subject to discussion and movement. Certainly, as ably demonstrated in the previous chapters, in all health-care settings the traditional boundaries between professional groups are being rethought and redrawn in response to professional development, local service needs, technological change and national policy objectives. However, much of this development to date has been ad hoc and uncoordinated. One of the United Kingdom Government's stated aims is to recruit and retain a workforce which has the capacity, skills, diversity and flexibility to meet the demands on the health service. However, professional politics and established power bases unfortunately often get in the way of coherent strategic approaches to workforce development. In this final chapter we put the case for a whole-system strategic approach to new role development.

Workforce planning

Unless the right number of suitably trained and experienced staff are available when and where they are required patients' needs will not be met. There has long been recognition that workforce planning is vital in the delivery of NHS services to meet the nation's health needs. The NHS Executive noted recently (1996) that 'the most important factor in the delivery of health services is the availability of an adequate number of well-motivated staff who are appropriately experienced, educated and trained. In order to ensure the supply of staff priority needs to be given to workforce planning, education and training, good employment practice and reward systems.'

The need for some form of forecast planning for the medical workforce has been accepted since the inception of the NHS. Since then there has been a series of reviews of the medical workforce on an almost 10-yearly cycle. The Medical Workforce Standing Advisory Committee has since 1992 been able to 'establish a continuing dialogue with the major interest groups and react to feedback in framing recommendations'. Other groups such as nursing, midwifery, the health-care professions (HCPs) and scientific and technical staff have a similar history. However, these predictions are often made in isolation from broader labour market issues. Workforce planning aims to find a balance between the supply of labour and the demand for that labour. However, this desire has to be set within a rapidly changing context in which attempts to balance supply and demand within existing professional structures will not necessarily address the changes required for service delivery and therefore new roles and perhaps even new professions will ultimately be required.

There has been considerable concern in the UK in recent years that there is a growing crisis in the recruitment and retention of clinical staff in all the health professions. The crisis is believed to be most acute amongst general practitioners (Leese & Young 1999), where it has been attributed to dissatisfaction with the NHS reforms, perceptions of increased workload, low morale and the move towards part-time working by an increasingly female workforce. The professional health-care workforce is dependent on output from university-based education programmes and migration from Europe and elsewhere overseas. Outflows from the workforce are related to retirement, emigration, career breaks and professionally qualified staff taking up alternative employment. Patterns of recruitment vary between specialties, with services such as the care of older people, psychiatry and learning difficulties having perennial recruitment problems. Patterns of retention also vary across the professional groups, with physiotherapists, for example, increasingly being employed in the private and independent sectors rather than the NHS.

The composition of the future professional workforce in health care will be predominantly female, even in medicine where the medical school intake is now over 50% female. This will increase the need for family-friendly employment practices and opportunities for part-time and flexible working. There are also significant geographical differences in the demand and supply of health professionals. London and other major urban centres in the South of England, which offer a wealth of alternative employment opportunities but labour under high costs of living, experience the most severe recruitment and retention difficulties evidenced by vacancy rates and the numbers of education places available through the universities' clearing systems. In the North of England and Wales, however, there are still significantly more applicants than places on pre-registration programmes in all of the health-care disciplines and a much more static workforce. Solutions must therefore be tailored to the needs of particular areas and there needs to be a general recognition that the health-care workforce operates in a series of distinct local labour markets rather than a single national market. Traditional notions of paid employment as having to be full-time and permanent are currently being challenged in many employment sectors. Similarly the notion of career structures as being necessarily linear and hierarchical seem increasingly less relevant in an era requiring a flexible and adaptable workforce (Davies 1995, Leese & Young 1999).

Professional power and influence

The definition of a profession has preoccupied sociologists for the last 40 years. The most influential analyses are those of Carr-Saunders & Wilson (1933), Talcott Parsons (1954) and, in relation to the profession of medicine in particular, Greenwood (1965) and Friedson (1970). Hopkins et al (1996) summarised the core attributes from these writings as follows: the possession of a body of specialised knowledge and altruistic service to clients. A long apprenticeship is therefore required to acquire the knowledge, entry to the profession is by examination of that knowledge and numbers are thereby controlled. As the knowledge is specialised, the profession holds that only the profession itself can be competent to judge whether good professional practice is being followed. From this follows the power of self-regulation. Altruistic service to clients implies that there are common values shared by members of the profession and a code of ethics. The profession itself also regulates departure from good professional practice according to the agreed values and ethics related to the profession. Professional status, however, depends on the willingness of society to grant the profession power and privilege in exchange for the profession's commitment to serve.

There has always been concern about interprofessional boundaries in health care and on occasion frank dispute. The archives of the Royal College of Physicians reveal an acrimonious and legally expensive war in which physicians and apothecaries attempted to define their separate responsibilities (Merret 1669, cited in Hopkins et al 1996). Even Florence Nightingale, despite her forthright reputation, said 'it is obvious that what I have done could not have been done had I not worked with the medical authorities and not in rivalry with them' (Nightingale 1855, cited in Mitchell 1984). In the clinical setting, doctors and nurses, according to Stein (1968), spend their professional lives playing a game in which the former repeatedly ask for and get advice and help from the latter but in such a way that the doctor's aura of omnipotence is preserved. Thus the rules require that the nurse make his or her recommendation in such a way that the idea appears to be initiated by the doctor. The doctor must listen for the recommendation, act on it and then carry on as though it had been his or her own idea to begin with. If the game is well played the doctor gains a valuable consultant, albeit one who is unheralded and not officially recognised. In this way nurses are only able to exert any influence over the process of care by manipulating individual doctors without really challenging the fundamental asymmetry of the power relationship. Stein et al (1990) reviewed the doctor-nurse game (Stein 1968) and plotted an increasing assertiveness amongst nurses. However, a series of short comments in the *British Medical Journal* in 1995 headlined 'Has nursing lost its way?' (Short 1995) suggests the pervasiveness of medical control, as we would be unlikely to see the work of medicine and doctors discussed in such an 'authoritative' and possessive way in a nursing journal.

Nevertheless, Hopkins et al (1996) suggest, in relation to medicine, that there has been an advancing erosion of professional control. They attribute this erosion in part to consumerism, the comparative routinisation of some technical skills, the multiplicity of new professions, attempts to control health-care costs through managed care and the reduction in junior doctors' hours which results in the need for greater numbers of juniors and substitution by nurses.

Regulation

The statutory regulatory bodies set the standards of practice for the professions they regulate. It is unclear whether or not the current system of regulating the health professions on unidisciplinary educationally based qualifications offers sufficient public protection. Consequently the role of the government health departments and employers is increasing in relation to determining fitness for practice for particular jobs and specialisms. Similarly devolution is encouraging a country-specific focus in workforce and service development priorities.

The United Kingdom Central Council for Nursing, Midwifery and Health Visiting (UKCC) in its evidence to the Fundamental Review of the *Nurses, Midwives and Health Visitors Act* (1998: 5), argued that the criteria for measuring the effectiveness of any regulatory system were that it should:

◆ be relevant to and ensure public protection
◆ secure the ownership and active participation of regulated professionals
◆ maintain public trust and confidence
◆ be achievable across an increasing range of health and social care settings
◆ be affordable for the organisations and individuals involved
◆ anticipate changes in health care and respond to them
◆ be fair and just in the results that it delivers
◆ deal with issues and cases expeditiously
◆ be adequately resourced and organised.

To retain public trust and confidence in the regulatory system standards that are based on demonstrated achievement in practice (competence-based standards) to ensure competence *in* practice of individual practitioners are likely to become increasingly important. The UKCC is leading the field in the development of regulatory mechanisms to enhance public protection. For example, it has developed a standard to distinguish those who are practising at a level significantly higher than that expected of registered nurses, midwives and health visitors. The 'higher level practice' standard identifies the specific outcomes against which practitioners will be assessed and which must be achieved by an individual for this attainment to be recognised by the UKCC and marked on the professional register. The standard is linked to a robust assessment process coupled with requirements for practitioners who have been recognised as practising at a higher level to update their knowledge and skills continually and provide evidence of their continuing competence. This is likely to assist good employment practices by the availability of a clear specification of this higher level of practice. Similar discussions are taking place in many of the other regulatory bodies.

The General Medical Council (GMC) in its guidance, 'The duties of a doctor' (1995), recognises the reality and value of teamwork and sets out the parameters by which doctors can delegate their work to other professionals. In this publication, the doctor is clearly seen as having a duty to ensure that any such delegation only takes place to an appropriately trained professional who is competent and willing to undertake the delegated task, and that the doctor retains full clinical responsibility. However, the GMC can only lay down the rules for doctors while other regulating bodies for nurses, pharmacists, physiotherapists and so on set the parameters within which these professions can function. Rather than the current myriad of professional bodies in health care it may be more appropriate in the future to develop a unified regulatory structure for all of the health professions linked to competence rather than completion of particular education programmes. Such a move is increasingly being demanded by consumers.

The National Consumer Council (1999) reviewed the self-regulation of professionals in health care. They found a patchwork of varying arrangements for different professions, differences in regulation between the public and independent sectors and legislation governing many regulatory bodies which has not caught up with changes in public demand or with current health-care practices. They noted that it is often difficult to find out what regulatory schemes there are and how they work to protect consumers. They concluded that regulation focused on individual professions in isolation may not adequately reflect contemporary needs and called for radical reform.

A question of competence

Competence should be central to any debate about the desirability or otherwise of new roles. Assumptions are an insufficient basis on which to make judgements about safe practice. Competence must be articulated and assessed, not presumed. The increase in educationally based qualifications held by practitioners does not necessarily imply competence, as we are all too tragically aware in the NHS. However, it is also important to consider that clinical competence in an area of care or intervention may not be the sole preserve of any one professional group. Within the framework of clinical governance NHS Trusts will need to make apparent the skills and knowledge that practitioners possess. Therefore, adopting a competence-based approach to new role development will offer an opportunity to make explicit the skills and knowledge required when delivering a clinical intervention and the appropriate staff group to undertake it.

The question of competence to undertake new roles is a growing concern for consumer organisations. For example, many national disease-specific organisations, such as the Parkinson's Disease Society and the cancer charities like Macmillan Cancer Relief and Marie Curie, along with small local charities such as BRACE in Bristol, are actively involved in evaluations of new clinical roles. Such evaluations should also to look beyond the posts to the organisational environment and even philosophy of service provision.

Consumers

The concept of patients as consumers has grown over the last decade. The essence of consumerism is that consumers should be able to get what they want rather than putting up with what providers choose to offer. For example, Hopkins et al (1996) suggest that the introduction of breast cancer nurses was driven initially by the demands of women rather than doctors. Acknowledging the issues articulated by Funnell in Chapter 7, consumers are increasingly articulating their individual and collective needs and wants on community health councils, as members of Trust boards and health authorities and within pressure groups such as patient associations. Therefore it is likely that consumers will represent a growing influence on the future shape and structure of the health-care workforce. The opening up of health-care knowledge, will rapidly change consumers' expectations of the services provided. As individual patients and consumer groups gain greater access to and understanding of health-care knowledge they will rightly begin to question the who, how, what and why of both interventions and services, including the personnel who deliver them.

Demography and changing patterns of need

Health-care need, and therefore health-care roles, are affected by changes in the structure of the population. The average lifespan is increasing and the birth rate is decreasing. The UK has a growing multiracial, multicultural population. The public, through government initiatives such as the 'Patient's Charter' is now encouraged to play an active role both in its own care and in deciding the future shape and composition of services and how they should be delivered. Patterns of disease and ill health are changing. There is likely to be an increase in chronic non-communicable disease, a growth in mental ill health, an increase in lifestyle-related problems due to obesity, drug and solvent misuse, and a growth in infectious diseases. Alongside these changes there is a growing interest in complementary therapies as an adjunct to mainstream health-care provision. The demand to provide culturally appropriate care that meets the health and demographic needs of the local population and ensures equitable access to services is vital.

Reconfiguring health services

The continuing push for a primary care-led NHS will shift the location and scope of services. This change in orientation and the shift in emphasis from secondary to primary care have tremendous implications for the education, roles and work patterns of health professions. The composition and make-up of the workforce will change, as Health Action Zones, Primary Care Trusts and 'Walk-in' services are established. Such community-based services are likely to continue to expand. These changes are likely to be assisted, as Davey has noted in Chapter 2, by the ongoing redefinition of the power and practices around the prescribing of drugs. For example, in acute care, Dowling et al (1995) found that an advanced neonatal practitioner (nurse) could provide almost total substitution for the clinical work of senior house officers, except of course for prescribing where there are legal constraints.

Education

A series of policy developments and professional initiatives since the 1970s has encouraged health-care professionals to work together in order to deliver high-quality care to individuals, groups and communities. Joint working, at best, is thought to cut down on duplication and overlap, prevent gaps in service delivery and help to clarify roles and responsibilities. Yet differences in educational backgrounds, financial structures, expectations, roles and systems can create barriers to mutual understanding. Health professionals have long been encouraged to develop shared goals and shared knowledge. Latterly this need to share expertise, pool knowledge and cross traditional boundaries has been portrayed not as a choice but as an essential ingredient of delivering high-quality health care. Interprofessional and multiprofessional education is being heralded as the means to achieve such collaborative practice. However, despite all these exhortations there has never been a coherent philosophy or strategy for operationalisation because funding streams and so on have remained steadfastly separate.

Increasingly the effects of the initiatives featured in 'The new NHS' (Department of Health 1997) relating to quality and clinical governance, the application of National Service Frameworks and the development of Primary Care Groups will affect the type of post-registration education that is needed. Working together: securing a quality workforce for the NHS (Department of Health 1998) emphasises the importance of continuing professional development and since April 2000 each local employer has been expected to have in place training and development plans for the majority of health professional staff. The new National Service Frameworks will require supporting education and training programmes. The provision of health care should not continue to be driven by the number of students trained and the content of that training; rather professional preparation and continuing education should be focussed on population needs.

Technology

Virtual reality technology is already affecting the education and training of surgeons and anaesthetists, and on-line health education will grow for both health-care professionals and consumers. NHS Direct and NHS Direct On Line will enable consumers to access health-care advice and health services directly. Although the impact of these developments will require a full and ongoing evaluation it is certainly clear that the advances in technology cannot be held back and will have a profound effect upon health-care provision and the composition of the health-care workforce.

There is little doubt that technology, both information and clinical, will play a role in changing how and who delivers health care. Technology will open up access to health-care information and will change the expectations of consumers and professionals alike. A growth of new scientific and technical professionals will accompany the developments in clinical technology. For example, in the fields of imaging and diagnostics there is considerable potential for the development of new roles. The regulatory framework, which to a certain extent currently determines the respective roles of the radiologist and radiographer, is firmly tied into the older technologies such as X-rays rather than the newer technologies such as magnetic resonance imaging. No one professional group will be capable of containing this change or holding on to an exclusive knowledge base to restrict its impact.

Cost

Hopkins et al (1996) note that it cannot be assumed that substituting a lower-paid health professional with the requisite skills to undertake tasks previously performed by a doctor will necessarily result in cost savings. Economic evaluations of new role developments are notoriously difficult. The ENRiP study (School of Health and Related Research (SCHARR) 1997) identified a number of issues in relation to costing the impact of new roles in acute care. Posts are often funded through soft money such as drug companies, project grants and charities. Often the systems of budgeting and resource allocation are generally such that service managers are unable to determine the opportunity costs of establishing such posts. For posts which are new, set-up costs could be calculated but many of these posts evolve from existing ones and in these cases costs are much harder to differentiate. Where training is required, this may be supported by the Trust or from other sources such as charitable trusts and replacement costs are not built in. Resources are also required for offices, equipment, support staff and clinic time. Other additional costs may be incurred for travel, telephone expenses and so on. Postholders are also believed to have a substantial impact on costs elsewhere in the service. These include increased patient attendance, the time cost of other staff attending training sessions that postholders run, increased or reduced pharmacy costs, and reductions in length of stay. Another complicating factor is that under the current contracting system purchasers pay for patient contacts with a doctor – regardless of who actually delivers the service – and service income is based on this premise.

Innovation in practice

Health-care professionals are human beings and as such will always test the boundaries of what is possible; there will always be a need for creative change in response to opportunity and demand in the delivery of services. The revelation that a theatre sister from Cornwall, had removed a patient's appendix established a continuing debate in the mainstream press about new role development. The *Sun* – a tabloid newspaper – even responded with a double page spread on how to remove your own appendix.

Nursing therefore provides a wonderful illustration of a profession which is constantly evolving and changing. Nurses have always adjusted the scope of their practice to meet changing health needs; for example, cannulation, defibrillation and even temperature-taking used at various times to be the exclusive preserve of registered medical practitioners. Changes in health policy that have encouraged a shift towards a primary care-led NHS, community care for people with mental health problems, and technological advances have all seen a response from nursing with the development of new roles.

Such changes have increased the decision-making authority of nurses. What was once unthinkable – nurses carrying out endoscopies, acting as specialists in diverse areas of care such as diabetes and behavioural therapy, running their own clinics in acute and primary care – is now becoming commonplace. Changes in regulation and the removal of restrictive role guidance that saw the introduction of 'The scope of professional practice' (UKCC 1992) encouraged nurses to take on new roles and activities to adapt to meet changing health-care needs. There are few tasks which nurses cannot now undertake legally. As particular tasks become more common – for example, cannulation, venepuncture and intravenous drug administration – they have become subsumed into the core skills expected of all registered practitioners.

As Walters notes in Chapter 5, the clinical nurse specialist roles in areas such as infection control, tissue viability, stoma care, continence and so on have existed informally since the early 1970s. Clinical nurse specialists were seen as experts in a particular area of care or with a particular client group, with post-qualification education and practice base firmly grounded in nursing. Nurse practitioners in primary care developed first in the late 1980s and offered an alternative service to that provided by general practitioners or filled gaps in service provision such as providing primary care to homeless people. They diagnose, refer, prescribe and provide complete episodes of care for clients with undifferentiated health problems.

In the 1990s posts emerged in secondary care with the title of nurse practitioner; these have frequently involved nurses giving care or performing tasks previously done by doctors. For example, advanced neo-natal practitioners are replacing junior doctors on the senior house officer rota in special care baby units. Surgical nurse practitioners run pre-admission clinics, clerk patients and organise theatre lists. Other nurse practitioners work across the primary/secondary care interface and prescribe within protocols for conditions such as hypertension and asthma, and now there are nurse consultant roles in the NHS (Department of Health 1999). The Secretary of State for Health, Alan Milburn, in his address to the Royal College of Nursing Congress, 2000, set out a ten-point challenge for 'liberating' nurses' talents, further evidence of the Government's committment to transforming health care roles.

Similar innovations are occurring across the spectrum of health-care professions, as contributors have illustrated in the preceding chapters, although interestingly they have tended not to occupy so many column inches in either the professional or the lay press. Each of these innovations will have consequences for the relationships between and even the continued existence of the various professions involved. For example, David et al (1982) found no significant difference between the outcomes of stroke patients treated by speech and language therapists and by untrained volunteers under the supervision of a language therapist.

Understanding systems

There are few areas where the need for mutual respect and cooperation between co-workers is as intense as in health care. To understand the world of health care we need to explore the relationships between its constituent parts. For example, as we noted earlier, much of the workforce planning in health care has occurred in separate professional groups and has been rather disconnected from service developments. However, anything that happens in one profession is bound to have an impact on the others. Therefore to encourage a strategic approach to change we need to explore the whole system and the relationships between its various elements in order to begin to understand the whole.

Health care requires a workforce that is flexible, adaptable and innovative so its exact composition will remain unpredictable. Within many sectors of the economy, workforces are having to adapt to meet the challenges of the global marketplace. An important characteristic of adaptive systems is that they learn. Using the example of a flock of birds Stacey (1996) illustrates that by each bird examining the behaviour of its neighbours and constantly changing its own the flock is able to fly in formation without crashing. This flocking behaviour has formed the basis of computer simulations, in which no one agent has control and no central programme determines the flocking strategy (Reynolds 1987). What occurred was a simple form of 'self-organising learning'. Therefore, from apparent randomness, successful outcomes can emerge. The connection between the behaviour of a flock of birds and the emergence of a new clinical role may not seem immediately apparent. However, new roles are often the consequence of the bottom-up, self-organising behaviour of an adaptive health-care system, that recognises a better way of doing things. It is evident that there has often been no central direction over that behaviour and in fact central control if too restrictive could constrain the essential adaptiveness that the system requires.

Many of the early influences that socialised individuals into professional groups can lock them into patterns and forms of practice that then become solidified regardless of their continuing appropriateness. Developing new roles requires professionals, managers and consumers to question their adherence to traditional ideas, structures and ways of doing things. Diversity and multiple ways of working are required. For professional groups who have a significant heritage and an established position within society this can be difficult.

Disturbance

Change is a form of disturbance for organisations and individuals alike. For organisational theorists such as Wheatley (1994) change is necessary to sustain the viability of organisations. Individuals, and, for that matter, organisations, need disturbance to learn and to develop the resilience for growth and renewal. Constantly expending energy to keep things the same in the face of change is tremendously wasteful. As we have seen in health care, all too often professions, organisations and individuals seek stability and equilibrium. Yet for Wheatley such a situation is a 'sure path to organisational death'. Stability may be seen as the point at which the capacity for change may be exhausted or extinguished. The evolution of new roles and the increasing demands placed upon health-care services are likely to be a continued source of disturbance. Stacey (1996) refers to the impact of such disturbance as 'creative destruction'. In his thesis it is suggested that groups evolve shadow systems and cultures that question the formal legitimate system and thereby create a process through which the organisation or system itself can evolve. Successful adaptive systems require disturbance to thrive, learn and develop resilience. The ways in which health-care professional roles continue to change illustrate complex adaptive systems in action.

Moving towards a strategic approach

The House of Commons Select Committee on Health (1999) has explored the wider workforce situation in the NHS; its recommendations reflect the complexity of the issues involved and highlight the importance of facilitating greater connectivity between professional groups and across sectors at local and strategic levels. The recommendations, summarised below, are a useful example of the need for a strategic, whole-systems approach to new role development in health care. The Committee recommended that:

◆ stronger formal links between the National Advisory Group for Scientists and Technicians (NAGST) and national professional bodies should be introduced
◆ there should be improved interaction between the medical and non-medical planning bodies
◆ there should be regular meetings between the Medical Workforce Standing Advisory Committee (MWSAC) and Regional Education & Development Groups (REDGs) to exchange information, discuss new ideas and develop plans
◆ there should be a major review of current planning procedures which should pay particular regard to their rationalisation and eventual replacement by an integrated planning system and joint training. Any new system should not only incorporate the national overview currently provided by the subgroup of the NHS Executive, but also actively promote a national strategy for workforce planning which, allowing for local conditions, brings a sense of consistency and cohesion

- ◆ the Department of Health should ask the MWSAC to look in more detail at the balance between specialist and generalist training for doctors in achieving a flexible medical workforce
- ◆ efforts are made to coordinate local initiatives and assess their strategic impact on future workforce numbers and that coordinated pilot studies are undertaken to assess the impact of altering the skill mix
- ◆ the proposed number of medical students be increased by a minimum of 1000 per year. This increase should be accompanied by a commensurate expansion in the number of senior doctors and consultants in order to provide for the necessary career opportunities and supervisory roles
- ◆ the Government urgently reassess its staffing figures to ensure an NHS workforce that is sufficient for requirements
- ◆ the Government consult with NHS employers and staff representative groups in order to establish a rigorous but fair system of efficiency appraisal
- ◆ the Department of Health consult with the Home Office and the Department for Education and Employment on the immigration status of and career opportunities for overseas staff
- ◆ the Government collate information from Trusts in order to allow them to formulate a specific recruitment and retention strategy for pharmacists, scientists and all of the HCPs as soon as possible
- ◆ health-care assistants working with nurses should be called 'assistant nurses' and be registered with the UKCC. Health-care assistants working with other professional groups should also be registered appropriately. Registration in such circumstances would provide professional motivation for the individual and would act as a necessary safeguard for the public who could then be assured that at all times care was being delivered by people whose competence was known and recognised
- ◆ overtime payments should replace undue reliance on agencies and the bank system should be used to cover unexpected shortages
- ◆ the NHS finance in full the relevant professional educational needs of its staff and extends current study arrangements
- ◆ the NHS move towards a single pay spine for all personnel. Terms and conditions should be negotiated nationally
- ◆ a single body should be established to review the pay of all NHS professionals.

The health service will continue to require reshaping to deal with changing patterns of need and demand which themselves reflect epidemiological, demographic and social changes within the population. The numbers of older people, for instance, will continue to increase, as will the prevalence of chronic diseases. These changes have already had an important influence on patterns of health-care organisation, reinforcing the move towards earlier discharge, more emphasis on primary care and care in the community, and greater teamwork in both acute and primary care. Consequently there is likely to be further innovation in the way that the 'work' is organised both within and between professions, and between professions and other groups of workers. Technological development is also certain to continue and possibly even to intensify with associated changes in the way some types of health care are delivered. It is probable that information technology and information systems will have a profound effect upon the way health care is delivered. There is also likely to be even greater specialisation. The scope and range of the UK Parliament's Health Select Committee's recommendations reflect the complexity that the health service faces in attempting to define, train, recruit and maintain a workforce that is able to meet these challenges. Its recommendations can thus be seen to span the diverse issues raised in this and previous chapters particularly in relation to recruitment and retention; the need for better regulation to ensure safe practice; the complex link between remuneration structures, costs and practice development; and the need for investment in education.

A global challenge

Whilst the focus in this book has been the United Kingdom, new clinical roles are developing in all health-care systems across the world and raising similar issues and tensions. Meaningful cross-national comparisons are difficult because even the nature and definition of many traditional health-care roles do not translate directly; for example, definitions of nursing, physiotherapy and occupational therapy vary between countries and health systems. The challenge of taking a patient-centred, strategic and proactive approach to new role development rather than a professionally led reactive one is, however, a global challenge. Within Europe, the 1986 *Single European Act* removed national boundaries in relation to the regulation and flow of capital, goods, services and people. This in effect created a Europe-wide marketplace for health professionals. At the moment, however, the only cross-national recognition of nursing and HCP roles is tied into initial registration and this reflects traditional roles rather than the new ones which are emerging (Keyzer 1994). Advanced and specialist practice roles also vary hugely across both North America and the Antipodes and across the states of the individual countries. This has implications therefore for flexibility and employment opportunities in an increasingly global health-care labour market.

Conclusion

Over the last decade many factors have accelerated new role developments in many health-care environments and across numerous specialties. These include an increasing evidence base around effective care delivery, governmental commitment to interprofessional working and new role development, advances in medical and other technologies, a heightened emphasis on improving service quality, developments in primary care, and changes in the medical workforce. Increasing attention to cost-effectiveness and value for money in association with difficulties in recruiting and retaining qualified staff in all disciplines has also had an impact. There is a need to improve the level of integration of the workforce planning process across the professions and with the business planning process at Trusts and Health Authorities. Comprehensive ongoing analysis of changing health and social care policy and the labour market will be crucial to determine future personnel needs.

The co-evolving processes of health need and workforce requirements, now more than ever, necessitate that we take a strategic 'whole-system' approach to the issue of new role development. Some of the fundamental assumptions that are currently held about existing roles, professions and boundaries need to be questioned. The current staffing 'crisis' in the NHS provides an opportunity to think the unthinkable and to let go of past constraints. Taking an organic view of this process may lead one to conclude that professional groups, like species, may become extinct over time as environmental conditions change. No single professional group can stand still in the face of the significant changes taking place in society's relationship with its health-care system. To survive these changes requires that the professions evolve and in that evolution they may become almost unrecognisable in terms of the nature of their role and function. In the longer term, the traditional conceptualisations of medicine, nursing, physiotherapy and so on are unlikely to be sufficiently flexible to address 21st century needs. We conclude therefore that professional groups are faced with a stark choice. They can either deploy their resources on defending their existing ground or embrace the macro-changes within the global health-care context and work strategically and proactively together with patients and other professions to create the changes in the workforce required to deliver appropriate and sustainable services.

REFERENCES

Carr-Saunders A M, Wilson P A (1933) The professions. Clarendon, Oxford
David R, Enderby P, Bainton D (1982) Treatment of acquired aphasia: speech therapists and volunteers compared. Journal of Neurology, Neurosurgery and Psychiatry 45:957–961
Davies C (1995) Gender and the professional predicament in nursing. Open University, Buckingham

Department of Health (DoH) (1997) The new NHS: modern, dependable (Cm 3807). Stationery Office, London

Department of Health (DoH) (1999) Making a difference: strengthening the nursing, midwifery and health visiting contribution to health and healthcare. Stationery Office, London

Dowling S, Barrett S, West R (1995) With nurse practitioners, who needs house officers? British Medical Journal 31:309–313

Friedson E (1970) Profession of medicine – a study of the sociology of applied knowledge. Dodd, Mead, New York

Greenwood E (1965) Attributes of a profession. In Zald M N (ed) Social welfare institutions – a sociological reader. John Wiley, New York:509–523

Hopkins A, Solomon J, Abelson J (1996) Shifting boundaries in professional care. Journal of the Royal Society of Medicine 89:364–371

House of Commons Select Committee on Health (1999) Third report. Stationery Office, London

Keyzer D (1994) European aspects of the nursing role. In Hunt G, Wainwright P (ed) Expanding the role of the nurse: the scope of professional practice. Blackwell Science, Oxford

Leese B, Young R (1999) Disappearing GPs. National Primary Care Research and Development Centre, Manchester

Mitchell J (1984) Is nursing any business of doctors? A simple guide to the 'nursing process'. British Medical Journal 288:216–219

National Consumer Council (1999) Self-regulation of professionals in healthcare: consumer issues. National Consumer Council, London

NHS Executive (1996) Education and planning guidance. EL 96(46)

Parsons T (1954) Essays in sociological theory, revised edn. Free Press, Glencoe, Illinois

Reynolds C (1987) Flocks, herds and schools: a distributed behaviour model. Computer Graphics 21:225–236. Cited in Stacey (1996)

Short J A (1995) Has nursing lost its way? Dual perspective. British Medical Journal 311:303–304

Stacey R D (1996) Complexity and creativity in organisations. Berrett-Koehler, San Francisco

Stein L (1968) The doctor–nurse game. American Journal of Nursing 68:101–105

Stein L T, Watts D T, Howell T (1990) The doctor-nurse game revisited. New England Journal of Medicine 322(8):546–549

United Kingdom Central Council for Nursing, Midwifery and Health Visiting (UKCC) (1992) The scope of professional practice. UKCC, London

United Kingdom Central Council for Nursing, Midwifery and Health Visiting (UKCC) (1998) The future of professional regulation. UKCC, London

Wheatley M (1994) Leadership and the new science. Berrett-Koehler, San Francisco

Index

Page numbers in *italics* refer to boxes and tables.